SACRAMENTO PUBLIC LIBRARY
828 "I" STREET
SACRAMENTO, CA 95814

12/2010

D0607833

THE
NO
OM
ZONE

THE NO OM ZONE

A NO-CHANTING, NO-GRANOLA, NO-SANSKRIT PRACTICAL GUIDE TO YOGA

KIMBERLY FOWLER

RODALE

The information in this book is meant to supplement, not replace, proper exercise training. All forms of exercise pose some inherent risks. The editors and publisher advise readers to take full responsibility for their safety and know their limits. Before practicing the exercises in this book, be sure that your equipment is well-maintained, and do not take risks beyond your level of experience, aptitude, training, and fitness. The exercise and dietary programs in this book are not intended as a substitute for any exercise routine or dietary regimen that may have been prescribed by your doctor. As with all exercise and dietary programs, you should get your doctor's approval before beginning.

Mention of specific companies, organizations, or authorities in this book does not imply endorsement by the author or publisher, nor does mention of specific companies, organizations, or authorities imply that they endorse this book, its author, or the publisher.

Internet addresses and telephone numbers given in this book were accurate at the time it went to press.

© 2010 by Kimberly Fowler

All rights reserved. No part of this publication may be reproduced or transmitted in any form or by any means, electronic or mechanical, including photocopying, recording, or any other information storage and retrieval system, without the written permission of the publisher.

Rodale books may be purchased for business or promotional use or for special sales. For information, please write to:
Special Markets Department, Rodale Inc., 733 Third Avenue, New York, NY 10017

Printed in the United States of America
Rodale Inc. makes every effort to use acid-free ♾, recycled paper ♻.

Photographs by Thomas MacDonald/Rodale Images
Illustrations by Karen Kuchar
Book design by Susan Eugster

Library of Congress Cataloging-in-Publication Data

Fowler, Kimberly.
  The no OM zone : a no-chanting, no-granola, no-Sanskrit practical guide to yoga / Kimberly Fowler.
      p.   cm.
  Includes index.
  ISBN-13 978–1–60529–674–6 paperback
  ISBN-10 1–60529–674–0 paperback
  1. Hatha yoga—Therapeutic use.   I. Title.
RM727.Y64F69   2010
613.7'046—dc22   2010011076

Distributed to the trade by Macmillan

2   4   6   8   10   9   7   5   3   1   paperback

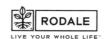

We inspire and enable people to improve their lives and the world around them

To anyone who has ever stood outside
a yoga class looking for a way in . . .

CONTENTS

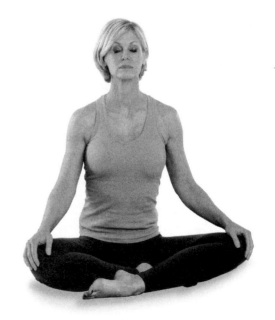

When I first started doing yoga back in 1983, it was to rehabilitate my body from a biking accident. I was hit by a car in a race outside of Dallas, Texas. I broke my collarbone, and actually bent the handlebars of my bike with my face—not pretty. After my injuries healed, I could not lift my arm higher than my shoulder. My goal was to get my body back to the point where I could return to the sports that I love. I was competing in triathlons at the time, so my sports were running, biking, and swimming.

Yoga was a means to an end for me. My physical therapist at the time was also a yoga instructor and would have me do yoga poses to help rehabilitate my shoulder. I didn't seek out yoga—it sort of found me. At the time, I never thought that I would become a yoga instructor, let alone develop my own style of practice. I just wanted to get back on the road as quickly as possible. It was a bonus that I stayed injury-free and could compete at a higher level than I ever thought possible. I remember, years later, walking into a yoga studio in Los Angeles, California, looking around the room, and thinking, "This just isn't for me." I knew the benefits of yoga and loved the feeling it gave me. But as an athlete with a type A personality, I watched everyone in the class twist themselves into pretzels and thought, "Why can't I do these poses?" To add insult to injury, the class started with the instructor saying, "Okay, everybody in handstands."

Well, I don't know about you, but doing a handstand in the middle of the room with a bunch of people all around me wasn't my thing. For one thing, I had broken my collarbone a few times. However, even if I hadn't suffered those injuries, I'm not sure I could do it. So I sat there thinking, "I'm never coming here again." At that point I saw a guy walk in who was obviously new to yoga. The telltale sign was that he walked in with his shoes on and didn't take them off. He didn't know what was going on, and I wanted to help him. I knew he would never come back and never do yoga again once he understood what would be expected of him in the class. I could so feel his pain. At that point I felt that I had to do something—it was a "Houston, we have a problem" moment. "How do I fix this? How can I help?" I thought. I never want someone to feel like that guy did in that yoga class. This book is for people like him.

My philosophy when it comes to yoga and, honestly, when it comes to most of the things I do in life, is to keep it simple. My motto in my classes is "safe, fun, and effective." Yoga is such a great exercise/workout for anyone; whether you are a couch potato, a weekend warrior, or a professional athlete, you will benefit from doing some yoga. I'm not trying to turn you into a member of Cirque du Soleil. You will see results—even if you just do yoga at home for 10 minutes a few times a week, you will see added muscle tone, flexibility, and possibly even an attitude adjustment. You don't have to give up your job, your sport, or anything that you love to do to go sit on a mountain and chant; that's not what this book is about. What it *is* about is showing you some simple poses that will take away muscle aches, alleviate pain, and help you calm your mind. I just want you to be able to live your life or play your chosen sport without injuries, aches, and pains. You might fall in love with yoga or you might not. What you will love is how it makes you feel when you're finished. I know taking a yoga class can be intimidating; I have been practicing for a long time, and it's still intimidating to me. That was the catalyst to starting my business, YAS Fitness Centers, creating my own style of yoga called Yoga for Athletes,® and writing *The No OM Zone*!

Yoga Keeps You Calm and Keeps You Going

This book takes a very practical, no-nonsense look at a 5,000-year-old practice and explains how it applies in the 21st century. I decided to call this book *The No OM Zone* because chanting "Om" during a class was one of the first things that turned me off yoga. If this happened to you, I am hoping you will give me a chance to reintroduce you to the amazing physical benefits of this practice. Among some of the benefits you'll discover: increased longevity; the ability to "stay in the game" no matter what your sport; and stress reduction, which in this fast-paced society is an extremely useful tool. With a simple "head-to-toe" approach, I break down the benefits of yoga for each major muscle group. I'll give you modifications and suggestions for common injuries and different sports. The goal is to keep you injury-free so you can "do what you love" for as long as you want. Some of the sports-related benefits of doing yoga are improved range of motion, increased muscle strength, and reduced post-workout soreness and muscle fatigue, which all add up to a big dose of injury prevention. Even if you're not an athlete, you can also experience improved posture, body awareness, circulation, energy level, relaxation, and stress relief. One of the main goals of this book is to get past the "yoga stigma," that is, it's a religion, a cult, or just for the chosen few who can twist themselves into pretzels. The goal of *The No OM Zone* is not just to expose the masses to yoga (because at this point, who hasn't heard of yoga?) but to teach you how to use yoga to your benefit even if you're not into all the chanting, Sanskrit, and granola.

Get Off the Couch and onto a Mat

This book will also prepare you to feel comfortable and confident, like a pro, before you even walk into your first yoga class. You'll find the answers to burning questions I get asked all the time, such as:

■ What should I wear, or not wear, to my first yoga class?

■ Should I buy a yoga mat?

■ How do you find the right class?

I'll also break down the different styles of yoga to help you identify what type of yoga best suits your personality and needs. Yoga is a multifaceted practice, and different styles produce different results. I'll help you find the one that's right for you.

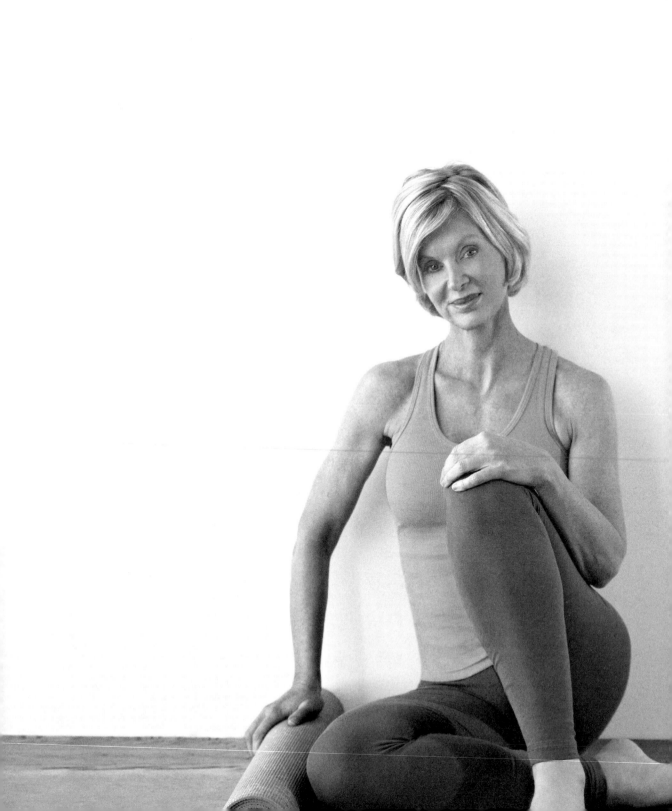

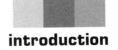

No Chanting, No Granola, No Sanskrit

The general attitude from people who don't do yoga, and even from some people who have tried a yoga class, is that it's a religion or a cult or only for people who can turn themselves into pretzels. Yoga can be very elitist, and off-putting, for the regular person on the street. This book is for those who have heard of yoga but haven't given it a try, or for those who have tried a class and thought, "This just isn't for me." Believe me, I can feel your pain, but I want you to give me a chance to change your mind. Don't worry, I'm not going to try to turn you into a pretzel—in fact, this is a "no pretzel zone." I don't want you to change your whole lifestyle, or to go sit on a mountaintop and chant! I just want you to be able to play your sport or live your life without injuries, aches, and pains.

What Is Chanting?

Chanting is the rhythmic speaking or singing of words or sounds, such as "Om," which is used as part of many religious rituals. It's very common in some of the more traditional yoga studios to chant in class. There is nothing wrong with chanting, if you subscribe to the spiritual side of yoga. However, for the purposes of this book, we are delving into the physical practice of yoga called Hatha Yoga.

Why No Granola?

One of the misconceptions about yoga is that it's for "hippies." Hippies are known for eating granola and wearing Birkenstock sandals. Yoga isn't just for hippies—it's for everyone.

This book takes a more practical interpretation of yoga. In most yoga books and Web sites, yoga is talked about as a cure for everything from migraines to menopause. We are going to take a look at each pose and try to decipher why the pose might "cure" you of an ailment. For example, Fish pose is said to cure anxiety and stress. Well, on a practical note, this pose releases the tension in your neck, thereby reducing your anxiety and stress—that makes sense, right? If you're familiar with the TV show *Dragnet* from the 1950s and 1960s, you'll remember that the lead character, Sergeant Joe Friday, used to say, "Just the facts, Ma'am, just the facts." That's what I'm going to give you. Just the facts.

What Is Sanskrit, What Is Yoga, and What Can It Do for Me?

Sanskrit is the Indo-Aryan language of Hinduism. A lot of yoga is still taught by using the Hindu language instead of English. Someone who is new to yoga may find it difficult to understand what the teacher is saying.

The yoga poses (also known as Asanas) in this book are broken down by body parts and muscle groups. Most yoga poses work numerous areas of your body. Let's say you are in the chest chapter and you are doing Downward-Facing Dog—this pose not only opens your chest but also helps stretch the back of your legs and strengthen your arms. Some sections in this book are going to be harder than others. Just as in the Olympics, I'm going to rate the "level of difficulty" for each pose, with 10 being the hardest. That way, if you are having a hard time doing a pose, you'll know that you are not alone.

Yoga is a full-body workout not only from head to toe but also from your inside to your outside. By that I mean that the poses in yoga not only work your muscles and joints but also affect your internal organs and nervous system. Yoga helps calm your nervous system by reducing the tension caused by stress. According to a 2005 study from Yale University School of Medicine, people who practice yoga at least three times a week may reduce their blood pressure, pulse, and risk for heart disease. Moreover, yoga improves heart health in both healthy individuals and those with diagnosed heart disease, says Satish Sivasankaran, MD, who conducted the study while training at Yale.

One of the main benefits I find from doing yoga is that it gives you more energy. You get so much more accomplished in a shorter period of time—who wouldn't want a little more energy to help you get through the day? I'm not going to ask you to spend hours upon hours a day doing yoga, because a little bit goes a long way. As I mentioned earlier, even doing just 10 minutes of yoga a few times a week will make a big difference. Your energy level will go up and your stress level will go down. If you have always been athletic but have been intimidated by yoga, even if it meant developing or maintaining flexibility, I get it. As a competitive athlete myself, I couldn't understand how the waif-like people in my yoga class could be so much better at it than me. I think that was the hardest part for me. I had to take the "competition" out of doing yoga. With yoga, you have to check your ego at the door. Don't expect to twist yourself into a pretzel the first time you try yoga. I've been practicing for nearly three decades, and there are still a lot of poses I continue to work on. That's the great thing about yoga—you will always be learning something new and challenging your body in new ways.

At the end of each chapter, you'll find quick yoga workout routines for a specific part of your body. You'll find workouts for your head, neck, shoulders, upper back, chest, arms, hands and wrists, core, lower back, hips, legs, knees, and feet and ankles. Don't worry, I will break down the poses so you know how to safely enter and exit each one. And as I mentioned earlier, you'll find modifications for each pose. I present an easier version and a harder version of the poses because some poses may be easy for you and some may not.

What If I Have an Injury?

Should you do yoga if you have an injury? Well, one of the main benefits of yoga is injury prevention. However, if you already have an injury, the first thing you should do is ask your doctor if it's okay to practice yoga. How do you recognize if you have an injury? If you are like most athletes, I'm willing to bet you ignore signs of injuries and write them off as soreness that will eventually go away. Pay attention! If you have any joint pain—that means pain in your knees, ankles, elbows, or wrists—or swelling, you need to be honest with yourself that these are signs of an injury. Before I start my yoga classes, I always ask about injuries (good instructors always do that). The first thing I check for is swelling in the area; if there is swelling, then I suggest that the student take the day off and see a doctor. Numbness in your body might be a sign of a pinched nerve; go see a chiropractor. You can bring this book with you to your physician and show him or her what you are planning on doing.

Here are some ideas on how to work other parts of your body while the injured area is recovering. Don't do any poses that directly affect the injured area. Let's say you tweaked your knee. You would want to skip the "yoga for the knee" chapter, but you can still focus on other areas of your body, like your arms, core, or upper back. So while your knee recovers, you could work on getting a "six-pack" or "yoga arms." In this situation you would do what are called "floor poses," as opposed to "standing poses" that work on your leg muscles and your knees. "No pain, no gain" does not apply in yoga—if it hurts, don't do it!

When it comes to injuries, my goal is to prevent you from getting injured in the first place. One of the main reasons yoga can help prevent injuries is its ability to prevent imbalances in your body caused by tight muscles. It's one of the few exercises that uses one side of your body independently of the other. In most workouts, the body will just compensate for the muscle imbalances. In each chapter, I will tell you "how the body part works." For instance, in Chapter 11, Legs, I discuss the anatomy of the legs so you can understand how the muscles of your legs work. Let me give you an example. When your quadriceps, the big muscles in the front of your thigh, are stronger than the hamstrings, the muscle in the back of your leg, a hamstring pull can result. This happens to a lot of runners—myself included, before I started practicing yoga.

Yoga versus Stretching

I'm often asked, "What is the difference between yoga and stretching?" Well, depending on how you "stretch," there may be no difference. In fact, in my "Yoga for Runners" workshops, I often hear someone say, "I already do that. I didn't know I was doing yoga." Most of the movements that we use when we are stretching come from yoga poses. But when you think of stretching, most of the time it's jerky, with a fast and forced movement, right? But when you think of yoga, you think of slow and controlled movements. I'm sure you have all seen runners grab an ankle and jerk their leg back and bounce it up and down. When I see that, I want to tackle the person and say, "Please stop! You are going to hurt yourself!" But I guess the tackling probably wouldn't go over very well, would it?

Unfortunately, most of the time when people stretch, they are trying to force their body to do something it's not ready to do. Yoga involves a lot more body awareness and attention to alignment. You *never* want to force yourself into a yoga pose. Athletes need to be especially careful to avoid this tendency since they, in general, are competitive, wanting to touch their toes *now*. Make sure you are warmed up before you do yoga or stretch.

What's the Mind-Body Connection About?

Yoga also has a mind-body connection, which I talk about in Chapter 1. This isn't normally part of stretching. The constant focus on the breath and the development of breath awareness gives you greater body control, which is necessary in all sports. The use of your breath in yoga will enhance your ability to carry oxygen to your muscles when you participate in sports. This translates into quicker reactions to unexpected situations encountered in running. For example, you might be chased by a pit bull or accidentally step into a pothole; unfortunately, I've experienced both. The breath work you do in yoga is the main reason for the "yoga bliss" (Chapter 1), that great feeling you get after a yoga class. After his first class, one of the guys in my class said, "Oh my God, this is like heroin. Yoga is my new fix." I have to say the comment threw me off for a second, but I think I get what he was trying to say. I hear similar comments from yoga novices. The feeling yoga inspires can be pretty great.

You Want Me to Stretch What?

Each chapter will go into some "anatomy." I'm not going to get too technical, and I don't want to bore you to death, but I feel it is always good to know some anatomy for any workout, whether it's yoga or any other sports activity. Yoga is all about "body awareness," but to know your body, you need to know how it works. When I am talking about "flexibility" in an area of your body, I am referring to what is called "range of motion," or how far you can bend that body part. Tight or stiff muscles can limit your range of motion. For example, my neck is stiff from writing, and that makes it hard for me to look over my shoulder right now. When it comes to anatomy in this book, I focus mostly on your muscles—when you are dealing with flexibility, you have little or no control over your bones, joints, ligaments, and tendons. We all know what bones are and what they do, but you might not know that ligaments connect our bones to each other and stabilize our joints; our muscles are connected to our bones by tendons.

As I mentioned earlier, the end of

QUICK-FIX TIPS

Similar to most workout routines, you want to do yoga on an empty stomach, or at least not right after you just had a big meal.

Some of the workouts in this book are harder than others, so each chapter will give you easier options and modifications for the poses.

It's always best to be warmed up first, so you can do the yoga workout routine after you run or work out at the gym. Personally, I like to take a hot bath before I do yoga at home.

Each yoga workout routine will start and end the same way. We will start with some breath work and end with an easy Spinal Twist pose and Corpse pose (also known as the Resting pose).

Remember: "No pain, no gain" does *not* apply to yoga.

If you have any injuries or other health issues, check with your doctor first to see if it's okay to do yoga.

each chapter features yoga for a body part workout routine. Each short workout will start with some breath work and end with the Corpse pose. Why? Well, I've already told you why breath work is so important, and Corpse is one of the most important poses in yoga. It seems so simple—as the name implies, you are just lying there. But if you are a type A personality, this may actually turn out to be one of your biggest challenges. You don't want to skip the Corpse pose, because it helps you to completely relax your body and your mind.

Okay, it's time to get started. You can start with the head and work your way down to the feet, or you may want to pick a specific part of your body, like your hips. Either way is good!

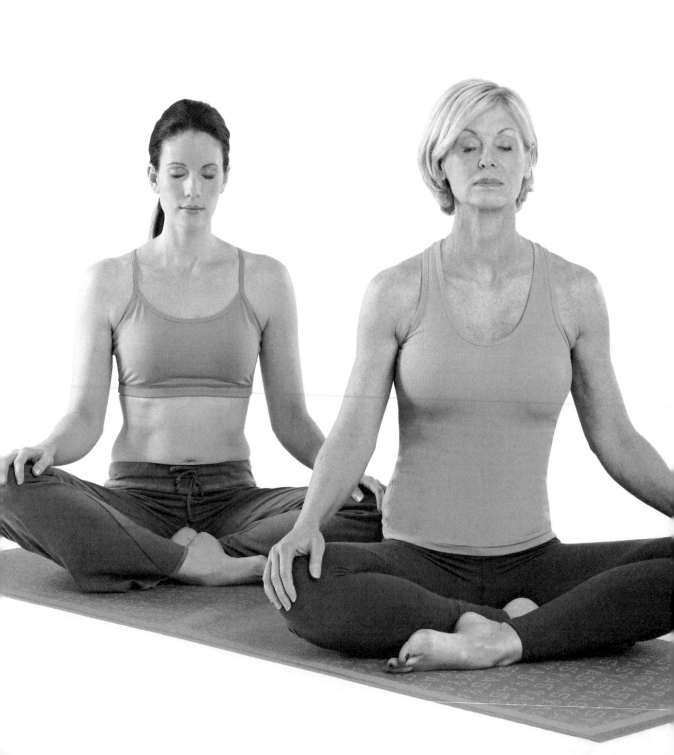

chapter 1

Head

Getting Out of Your Head

So when you think of yoga poses for the head, what comes to "mind" (pardon the pun)? Probably Headstand, right? Don't worry, I'm not going to ask you to stand on your head. Well, at least not *yet*! Headstand is an advanced pose and shouldn't be done until you have been practicing yoga for a while. We are going to first focus on the mind-body connection, which includes what is called "breath work." Breath work is a great place to start because it is one of the main components of yoga that differentiates it from other forms of exercise or stretching. Some types of yoga, like Kundalini, are actually more about breath work than about doing the physical poses.

Now some of you may think, "I already do some stretching. Why do I need to do yoga?" Well, yoga is more than stretching, mainly because of its mind-body aspect. The mind-body connection makes yoga a more appealing workout for me because I'm getting two for one. When we think of "fitness," most of the time we just think of our bodies. In yoga, as with life, the mind and the body are connected—as any athlete knows, the mind can actually help your physical performance. I have always believed in the power of the mind over the body.

So how does yoga connect the mind and the body? Well, one of the main ways yoga affects the body, and in particular the head, is through the use of breath work. In a yoga class, the teacher will usually start and end each class with breath work. The practical application of breath work is that it will help with just about any sport, be it running, cycling, basketball, or swimming. All of these activities take good breath control, but a large part of athletic ability and performance is mental. I think running a marathon is mostly mental. When you go into "the zone" in sports it means you exceed your normal physical abilities; this is when the mind and the body connect. Part of this is caused by controlling your breath, which keeps your body and mind operating at peak efficiency. Yoga uses your mind to help you build a healthy body, and in return it makes you an all-around better athlete/parent/boss/person in general.

While every chapter in this book addresses muscle group–specific yoga poses, the mind-body connection is a part of each of these. Every section will start with a little breath work, which brings the mind and body together. That way it becomes a more "mindful" workout. It's not like lifting weights; you don't just grab a dumbbell and go at it without thinking. You want to stay focused on what you are doing to the point where yoga becomes a moving meditation.

So what exactly is meditation? Well, as with yoga, there are a lot of different schools of "thought," no pun intended, on meditation. I don't know about you, but I find that life can be pretty stressful. We "go go go" from day to night. Plus we are overloaded with information, almost to the point where we cannot think at all. So I gravitate toward things that are simple, straightforward, easy to do, and, of course, effective. In this chapter, I go into the different forms of meditation so you can see which one you like or will work best for you.

I started meditating because when I was taking classes, most of the yoga instructors would talk about meditation. Being the typical type A personality, within the first month of starting yoga I not only took my first yoga teachers' training class but also a course in meditation. There are tons of different theories, so I tried a bunch of different practices. I did what I consider one of the more "extreme" versions of meditating called Vipassana.

That's where you sit for 10 to 12 hours a day for 10 days straight and just meditate. It's a silent meditation, and for me the silence was the best part. I was a lawyer at the time—just the thought of not having to talk to anyone for a week was *heaven*. Now, the sitting for 10 to 12 hours part was a whole other ball game! I can still remember it as if it were yesterday. You just sit and don't move at all. The only thing l could think about for 10 hours a day was, "Oh my God, my ass hurts." I know, I know, it's not very enlightened of me.

Vipassana was originally used for drug addicts in India; they would be locked up in a box for 10 hours a day. I took the course in northern California, and though they didn't lock you up, I did get blocked in. Someone parked behind my car, which, unfortunately, I found out when I was trying to escape in the middle of the night. How embarrassing to admit that! But I couldn't ask someone, "Can you please move your car so I can sneak out?" It was a silent retreat, which means even if I asked, no one would answer. So I was forced to stay there the full 10 days.

The type of meditation that I found was best for me—Ms. Type A—was Transcendental Meditation (TM). This practice became famous when the Beatles started practicing it back in the 1960s. It is very logical and is backed up with scientific proof that it helps reduce stress and lower your blood pressure. Celebrities such as Russell Simmons and Jerry Seinfeld use TM to help them relax and get focused. It gives you the sense of "restful alertness," and who wouldn't want that? In a stressful society, where we feel tired all the time, meditation and yoga calm you down and give you energy at the same time. I know none of us have any extra time, and I know I am asking you to find the time to do yoga and meditation. But the benefits you will get from it—by having more energy, thinking clearer (no more "brain fog"), and decreasing your stress—will, I promise you, be well worth the 10 to 20 minutes per day.

How Does the Head Work?

Your head weighs around 11 pounds. So let's start from the outside of your head, aka the skull. There are 22 bones in the skull. The upper part, the cranial skull, protects the brain and is composed of eight bones. The other 14 bones make up the structure of your face. The brain itself is extremely complicated and accounts for about 2% of your total body weight. However, it takes 20% of your blood supply to keep it functioning. When you sleep, your body is resting but your brain stays active.

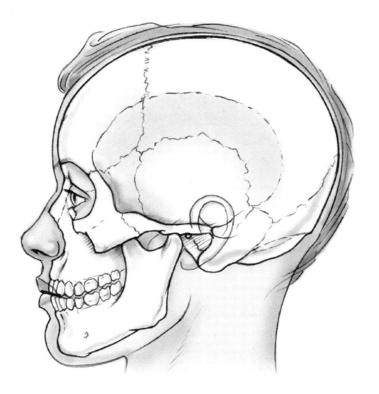

Common Injuries/Issues with the Head

Stress: Probably the number one comment I get from my students who start to do yoga is, "I don't feel stressed out any more." So how does yoga help with stress relief? We all deal with stress, and I'm sure you have heard of the "fight or flight" response—that's when your adrenaline starts pumping through your body. Breath work helps calm your body. Think about it. What do you do when you get stressed or angry? You stop breathing, right? As you are reading this, I want you to take a deep breath in through your nose and then exhale it out through your mouth. Repeat this a few times and I promise you that you'll start to feel a little calmer. I live in Los Angeles, California, so I find myself using this technique when I am driving; if you have ever driven in LA you know what I am talking about! Once you learn breath work, you can use it all throughout your day. I have students who tell me that instead of going into "road rage," they thought of my yoga class, took a deep breath, and found themselves calmed. They heard me in their heads saying "breathe." Try this and you'll be amazed by how quickly you will calm down.

Yoga helps with stress in numerous ways—not only by calming your mind but also by making your body strong, flexible, and resistant to injury. Injuries can be stressful for anyone because they take you out of the game and they require healing.

We all experience stress in our daily lives from several different sources: Jobs, relationships, and finances are at the top of the list. Stress can take a significant toll on you both physically and emotionally. And, as most doctors will tell you, stress manifests itself in many different ways:

- Headaches/migraines
- Frequent colds or flu
- Sleep disorders
- Anxiety
- Not feeling clearheaded (brain fog)
- Feeling frustrated
- Lowered libido

Stress in smaller doses can actually give you energy, makes you more alert, and helps you focus. Many people work well "under pressure," and this type of stress can actually be a good motivator. When you are at this level of stress, you might feel pumped up or wired. As the level of stress increases, it becomes harder to cope with certain situations and you begin to feel stressed out, burned out, and tired all the time. It's important to be aware when this begins to happen so you can find positive and productive ways to deal with the stress. We all handle stress differently, and the symptoms of stress manifest themselves differently in each person. Yoga iş an amazing equalizer and a definite "stress buster."

Migraine headaches: From what I have read about migraine headaches, they seem to be caused in part by changes in the level of a chemical called serotonin. Serotonin plays many roles in the body, and it can affect the blood vessels. When your serotonin levels are high, blood vessels constrict. When serotonin levels fall, the blood vessels swell. It's this swelling that can cause pain or other problems. For those of you who have had one, you know the pain of a migraine headache can be intense. It can actually get in the way of your daily activities. Yoga can help relieve migraines by bringing blood supply back to your head and releasing tension in your neck (see Chapter 2, Neck). Migraines aren't the same in all people. Possible symptoms of migraines include the following:

- Intense throbbing or dull aching pain on one or both sides of your head
- Nausea or vomiting
- Blurred vision or blind spots
- Sensitivity to light, noise, or odors
- Feeling tired or confused
- Stiff or tender neck
- Light-headedness
- Tender scalp

Vertigo: Vertigo is the feeling that you or the room around you is moving or spinning. There are numerous causes for vertigo, and yoga can help with the stress-related ones.

Poses to Help Your Head

Meditation

Benefits: Meditation is a big part of the practice of yoga. One of the benefits from meditating is that you don't need as much sleep—you can get by with 5 hours of sleep a night instead of needing 8 to 10 hours—and of course you'll still feel great. I read once that Deepak Chopra gets up at 4 a.m. I thought, well, if it's good enough for him, it's good enough for me, so I started getting up at 4 a.m. People think I'm strange when I tell them that I get up that early. I don't tell them it's because I meditate; I just say, "I'm on East Coast time." Since I live in Los Angeles, everyone says, "Oh, that's cool." I guess that's better than people thinking I'm a weirdo!

One of the most fascinating facts I found on meditation is that after the age of 35, our brain cells start to die off at a rate of 100,000 per day, and they don't come back—scary! Meditating will help reduce that rapid rate of declining brain cells. That little fact alone would get me into meditating if I didn't practice already. People who meditate "regularly," meaning daily, not just once a year, start to develop this calmness. I can walk into a room and know who meditates and who doesn't. If you don't believe me, just try it for a month and see what happens.

Now, the same principles apply as those we talked about in the introduction: No one is perfect, and doing a little is better than not doing it at all. Don't judge yourself; don't think, "I'm not meditating correctly or doing it right, I don't feel enlightened after meditating for 5 seconds, what's wrong with me?" I'm not judging you for feeling that way—

our society rewards people who take on high-stress jobs, the overachievers. We want to make sure every minute counts. I want you to do yoga and meditation so that you use your stress in a positive way by fine-tuning your mind, so it works efficiently and you are able to concentrate and focus. You can also hit your "zone" in meditation, as you do in sports. It's called Samadhi, a Buddhist term that means a higher level of concentrated meditation. Samadhi is considered a precursor for enlightenment—that is, Nirvana, also known as "yoga bliss." When athletes are in "the zone," they have reached their peak performance. The same with meditation: Your mind is thinking quickly, sharply, and accurately. This happens because meditation reduces stress, helps reduce headaches, energizes you, and calms your body all at once.

Types of Meditation

All meditation techniques can be grouped into two basic approaches:

■ **Concentrative meditation** actually focuses your attention on the breath, an image, or a sound (mantra) in order to still the mind and allow a greater awareness and clarity to emerge. TM or Transcendental Meditation, which we talked about earlier, would be classified under this type of meditation. The easiest form of concentrative meditation is to sit quietly and focus the attention on your breath. When you do yoga, there is a direct correlation between your breath and your state of mind. For example, when you are anxious, frightened, agitated, or distracted, the breath will be shallow, rapid, or uneven. On the other hand, when the mind is calm, focused, and composed, the breath will tend to be slow, deep, and even. Focusing the mind on your inhalation and exhalation provides a natural and easy way of meditating. As you focus your awareness on the breath, your mind becomes absorbed in inhalation and exhalation, or at least that's the goal. As a result, your breathing will become slower and deeper and the mind will become calm and aware.

■ **Mindfulness meditation** involves opening one's attention to become aware of continuously passing sensations and feelings, images, thoughts, sounds, smells, and so forth without becoming involved in thinking about them. You just sit quietly and witness whatever goes through the mind, not reacting or becoming involved with thoughts, memories, worries, or images. I personally find this more challenging because I want to engage my thoughts—you know, talk to myself, which I have to admit I do all the time. The goal of this type of meditation is to gain a calmer, clearer, and "nonreactive" state of mind.

Meditation Pose

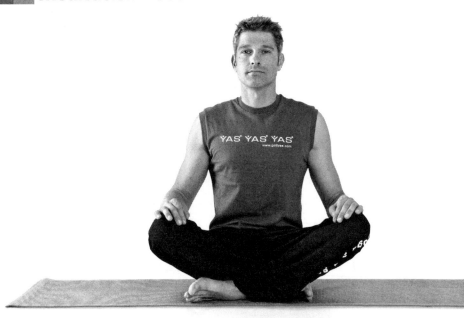

QUICK-FIX TIP **If you have pets, lock them out of the room. For some reason, when you meditate your pets will gravitate to you. My dog Lucky tries to sit on my lap whenever I go to meditate—she is an 80-pound golden retriever, so it's a little hard to breathe when she is sitting on top of me. That's why I meditate in a chair instead of the floor. If you are having problems sleeping, try meditating at night, before you go to bed, to help clear your mind. It's hard to fall asleep when your head is buzzing with the stock market, the economy, and housing prices. Meditating at night is one answer; another is "Don't watch the news before you go to bed!!"**

How do you get into this pose?

- Find a quiet place in your house to sit— bedrooms are usually your best bet.

- Select a word or mantra. Choose a word that inspires you.

- Sit comfortably in a chair or on the floor. If you are on the floor, it's a good idea to sit up against a wall to keep your back straight.

- Sit in an easy cross-legged position.

- Sit up straight, close your eyes.

- Bring your hands on your thighs; take a minute to scan your body.

- If your shoulders are tight, relax them.

- Repeat your mantra.

- Sit for 5 to 20 minutes. You can start with 5 minutes if you want; just do what you can at first. After sitting for 5 minutes, take a deep breath and just let it go.

"Yoga for the Mind" Workout Routine: 5–20 Minutes

Find a place to sit in your house quietly; it can be a chair or the floor. If you decide to sit on the floor, sit up tall in a cross-legged position, with one leg in front of the other. If this is challenging, then lean your back up against a wall. Bring your hands on your lap or your thighs.

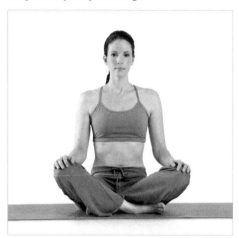

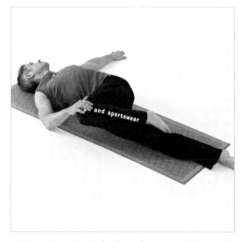

BREATH WORK Sit up tall and close your eyes. We are going to take a minute to center your body and get you focused on your head or focus on getting "out of your head." Take a deep breath in through your nose and exhale it through your mouth. Repeat this two more times, and each time try to hold your breath for a few moments before you exhale.

Pick a word, which will be your mantra. Think of something that is inspiring to you. This will help focus your mind if thoughts come up; just go back to thinking of your word. At first your mind might be all over the place, with thoughts of work, paying your bills, your kids, even things as simple as what you need to buy at the grocery store. Believe me, it does get easier the longer you do it. It may take a week or two to be able to sit longer than 5 minutes. If you want, you can set an alarm clock—that's what I did when I first started. Try not to have one eye on the clock; keep your eyes closed. When you are finished, take a few seconds to notice how you feel. I usually have a pen and some paper close to me when I meditate. You may want to do this too because you may have all types of great ideas come to you!

EASY SPINAL TWIST Let's end your meditation with an Easy Spinal Twist to release your lower back from sitting. Come down to the floor on your back and then hug your knees into your chest. Bring your left knee into your chest and move your right leg straight out on the floor. Bring your left knee across your body while keeping your shoulder blades on the floor. Look over your left shoulder to complete this twist. Hold for 20 to 30 seconds, then hug both knees into your chest. Switch sides: Right knee comes into your chest, right leg goes straight. Bring the right knee across your body and look over your right shoulder to complete the twist on the right side. Take a second to notice the difference from one side to the other. Hold for 20 to 30 seconds, then bring both knees into your chest. Now you are ready to take on your day!

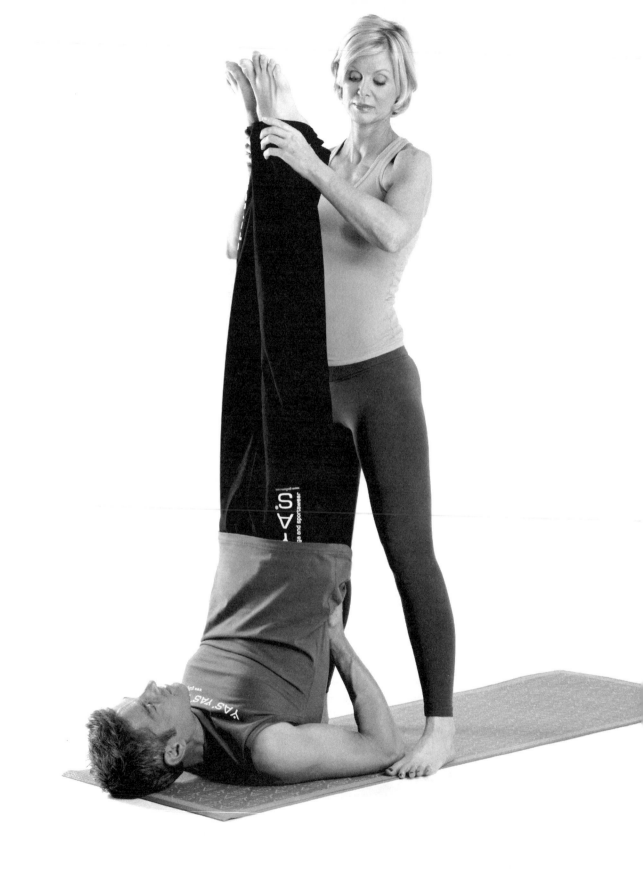

chapter 2

Neck

What's That Pain in the Neck?

In one way or another, most yoga poses deal with your neck as an extension of your spine. So if you are practicing yoga, you are most likely helping your neck relax and become more supple. Most of us are at our computers all day with our heads lurched forward. This hunched position causes the muscles in the back of your neck to get tight and short. Yoga can help loosen your neck muscles by stretching them, which will help you get rid of tension. As you already know from Chapter 1, the average head weighs about 11 pounds and your neck has to support it all day. It's like walking around balancing a bowling ball on top of your neck. Many of the issues you might have with your head, such as headaches, come from something as simple as tension or tightness in your neck muscles. Full disclosure: While writing this book, I became so stiff that my neck started

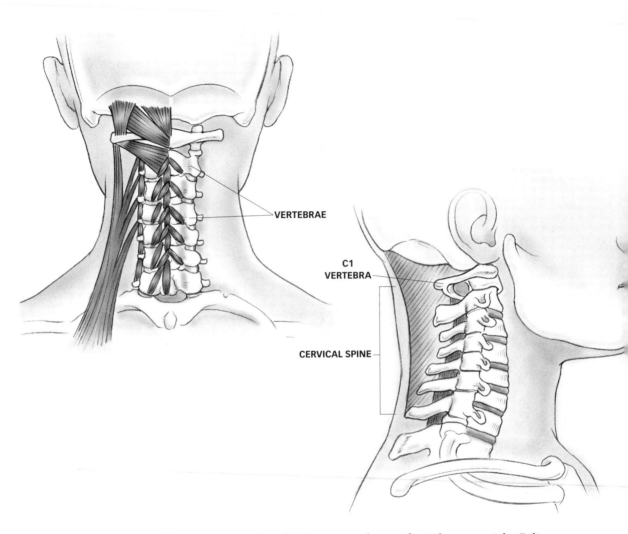

VERTEBRAE

C1
VERTEBRA

CERVICAL SPINE

to spasm. It was driving me crazy. One day I just sat and wrote for 16 hours straight. Believe me when I say "I can feel your pain!"—even as someone who has practiced yoga for some 20 years! Since I didn't have the time to take a class, I did the 10-minute yoga for your neck routine instead. It's really helped, and I'm not just saying this because it's my book!

How Does the Neck Work?

Most neck pain starts in the top part of the neck called the cervical spine. The cervical spine supports the head with C-shaped bones. The mobility in your neck comes from seven bones that interlock, which are called your vertebrae. I'm sure you have heard of a part of your neck that chiropractors or doctors might refer to as "C1 to C2," et cetera. The C1 vertebra is a ring-shaped bone that supports and balances the skull. The cervical bones—the vertebrae—are smaller than other spinal vertebrae. The purpose of the cervical spine is to contain and protect the spinal cord, support the skull, and enable diverse head movement. This forms the flexible joint, which lets you nod your head "yes" and shake your head "no." Each vertebra allows a relatively small amount of movement, but together they let you rotate or move your head to the side and to move it forward and backward. There is also a complex system of ligaments, tendons, and muscles that help to support and stabilize the cervical spine. Ligaments work to prevent excessive movement that could cause serious injury. Muscles also help to provide spinal balance and stability and enable movement. While this isn't the complete anatomy of the neck, it gives you the basic idea of how it works.

Common Injuries/Issues with the Neck

Muscle spasm: Muscles go into spasm when all the fibers within the core of a muscle contract simultaneously. This most commonly occurs when you suddenly move or overextend a tense, tight muscle that hasn't been properly prepared for the movement. Neck muscles are often tight and tense, and that's why they are more vulnerable to becoming overstressed by small movement. Muscle spasms are caused by:

- Stress
- Sitting for long periods of time (at a computer or during driving or flying)
- Injury
- Overuse
- Postural problems

Symptoms include:

- Intense pain
- Neck stiffness
- Burning or pins-and-needles prickly feeling

Muscle strain: Muscle strain in the neck is caused by a tear in the small muscle fibers that slide over one another when you move your neck. Sometimes this tear can be microscopic, or can cause bleeding or overstretched fibers. Muscle strains are caused by:

- Overuse
- A sudden and strong impact, including whiplash and contact sports
- Too much muscle tension (e.g., lifting heavy weights)

Symptoms include:
- Pain
- Neck stiffness
- Headache
- Dizziness
- Burning or pins-and-needles-prickly feeling

Whiplash: Whiplash is an injury to the neck caused when the neck and head are thrown suddenly backward and then forward upon impact, as in a car crash. The impact forces the neck and head beyond their normal range of movement, causing tissue damage and pain. Whiplash is caused by:

- Car accidents
- Sports injuries
- Blows to the head from a fall

Symptoms include:
- Headache
- Pain in the shoulders
- Pain between the shoulder blades
- Pain in one or both arms
- Fatigue
- Dizziness
- Vision problems
- Poor concentration or memory
- Neck pain/stiffness
- Tight and/or sore muscles
- Tenderness in the muscles
- Lower back pain

■ Sleep disturbance

■ Loss of motion in the neck

Stinger: A stinger is an injury that affects the nerves in the neck and arms. It happens when the neck is suddenly forced to rotate or tilt excessively. As with whiplash, impact can also cause a stinger. You will know if you have a stinger because you'll feel burning or stinging in the area of the neck. This usually happens in contact sports such as football, but it can happen just from turning your head too quickly. Stingers are caused by:

■ Sports injuries

■ Quick movement of the neck toward the opposite shoulder

Symptoms include:

■ Intense pain

■ Tingling or burning sensation

■ Numbness or weakness in arm or hand

The neck, though small, is a complicated area of the body, so unfortunately there are lots of ways to injure it. The preceding lists mention just a few of the more common ones. The following yoga poses will help alleviate tight neck muscles. Remember, if you have any neck injuries, talk to your doctor before you do any workouts.

POSES TO HELP YOUR NECK:

1. Bridge pose

2. Plow pose

3. Shoulder Stand pose

4. Knees to Ears pose (aka, Deaf Man's pose)

5. Fish pose

Bridge Pose

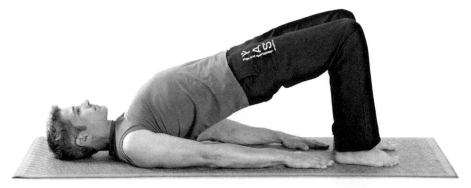

Benefits Bridge is a backbend that opens the front of your body (mostly your chest); it also elongates and stretches the muscles in your neck. So this pose stretches your chest, neck, and your spine and is said to be a great stress reducer. This makes sense because we hold a lot of our stress in our neck, shoulders, and upper back. Because Bridge pose strengthens the back of your body, opens the front of your body, and stretches the back of your neck, it's an effective preparation for Shoulder Stand and a great pose for keeping your neck in good shape. The main physical limitations that get in the way of "building your Bridge" are shortness in the front of your body, stiffness or injury in the neck, and weakness in the back of your body. Don't worry, the more you do Bridge, the sooner you will see these limitations disappear.

The degree of flexibility in your spine comes into play here, too. Typically, a stiff middle and upper back will stay rounded in a hump even as the neck and lower back go into the backbend. If your upper back stays rounded like this when you try to do back-bending poses such as Bridge or Camel, then the lower back will compensate by overarching or hyperextending. When the lumbar spine extends too much, it becomes vulnerable to painful compression

and short, achy lower back muscles. Ideally, you want the whole back working in Bridge pose.

So what keeps the upper back-neck area from bending backwards in Bridge pose?

It could be an injury or arthritis in your neck that limits your range of motion. However, normally the neck stays rounded because the muscles of the front body and connective tissue around the spine and rib cage are short and tight. These muscles include the pectorals, which run across the front of the chest; the rectus abdominus, which runs straight up the middle of the abdomen; and the front lower ribs and the obliques, which we will go into in the core/abs chapter.

Consider the shoulder position in Bridge pose

As your hips and lower back lift off the floor and the arms press down into the floor, the shoulders move toward each other. Assuming that the shoulder joint isn't injured, the muscles that limit extension are the same muscles that perform flexion: the upper portion of the pectoralis major, which covers the upper front chest, and the anterior part of the deltoid muscle, which forms the cap covering the shoulder joint. By stretching the pectoralis major and the anterior deltoid, you'll increase the range of motion in shoulder extension, which will enable you to lift your rib cage higher and open your chest more in Bridge.

There are a few ways to do this while you are at work sitting at your desk. Start by interlacing your fingers behind your back, standing or seated, with the cup of the palms facing upward. As you straighten your elbows, move the shoulder blades down away from your ears and back, to open your chest. To increase the stretch, move your hands away from your lower back without overextending your lower back or letting your shoulders roll forward. If your shoulders roll forward, you'll collapse and drop your chest, which you don't want to do in Bridge.

How do you get into this pose?

- Lie on the floor.
- Bend your knees.
- Bring your feet flat on the floor.
- Bring your feet hip-distance apart and parallel.
- Keep your knees in line with your heels.
- Reach down with your fingertips to see if you can feel your heels. If not, then walk your heels a little closer to your body.
- Press your weight into your feet to lift your hips up toward the ceiling.
- Keep your thighs parallel.
- Bring your arms underneath you and try to clasp your hands together. (Don't worry if you can't do it at first.)
- Roll your shoulder blades toward each other.
- Hold this pose for 45 seconds to 1 minute, then release.

QUICK-FIX TIPS Try to get your chest to your chin and your hips to the ceiling. Over time, as you're able to lift the chest more, the muscles in the back of your neck will stretch and lengthen, which can be quite a relief if you have short, tight muscles. If you feel pain during or after Bridge pose, try placing a folded blanket, or even two, under the arms and shoulders, with your head on the floor and your neck curving over the edge of the blanket. This should reduce any strain on your neck.

- Roll slowly back to the floor.
- Repeat two more times.

Modify the Pose Bring your hands to your lower back for support.

Level of Difficulty On a scale of 1 to 10, I would give this pose a 6.5. Depending on the flexibility of your neck, chest, and shoulders, it might be harder or easier for you.

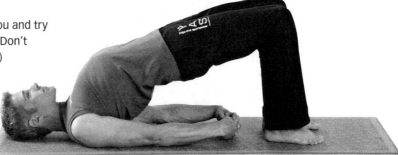

Plow Pose

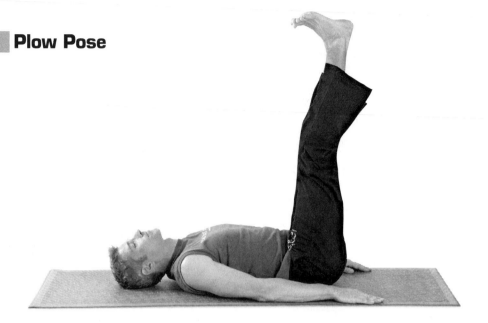

Benefits Plow pose is a great stretch for your neck but also for your entire back. This pose is another one that claims to cure, well, everything. Let's break down some of the claims for this pose. Here are some of the more popular ones: *Calms the brain*—Well, as an inversion (see discussion of Shoulder Stand position later in this chapter for an explanation of inversion), it involves bringing your legs over your head and letting blood go to your head, which helps with migraines. So I guess you can see why this pose might calm the brain—we saw in Chapter 1 just how much blood the head needs to function. *Stimulates the abdominal organs and the thyroid gland*—When you get into this pose you may see why this would be the case. How could it not stimulate your internal organs and your thyroid gland? *Stretches the shoulders and spine*—This one is a given. *Helps relieve the symptoms of menopause*—Hmm, not so sure about this one. *Reduces stress and fatigue*—I can see how it decreases stress because it opens the neck muscles. As for fatigue, well, it's an inversion, bringing

blood to your head. *Therapeutic for backache, headache, infertility, insomnia, sinusitis*—Most of this I would agree with, except for the infertility part. I'm not sure how that would be the case from just looking at the pose from a physical aspect.

How do you get into this pose?

- Lie on the floor.
- Bring your legs straight up in the air toward the ceiling.
- Bring your arms alongside your body with your palms down.
- Press into your hands to lift your legs over your head.
- If your legs do not touch the ground behind you, then bring your hands to your back to support your back.
- If your feet do hit the ground, then do what you did in Bridge pose, by clasping your hands together and trying to roll your shoulder blades toward one another.

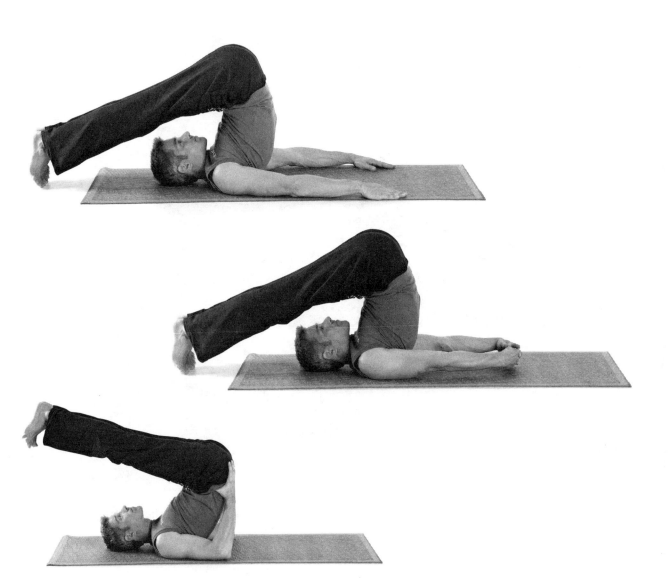

Modify the Pose Keep your hands on your lower back, and do not drop your feet to the floor.

Level of Difficulty A solid 7.

QUICK-FIX TIP **Do not turn your head once you are in the pose because it will strain your neck muscles. If you take a yoga class, you might be tempted to look around the room to see what everyone else is doing. DON'T! You are doing this pose to help your neck, not hurt it.**

Shoulder Stand Pose

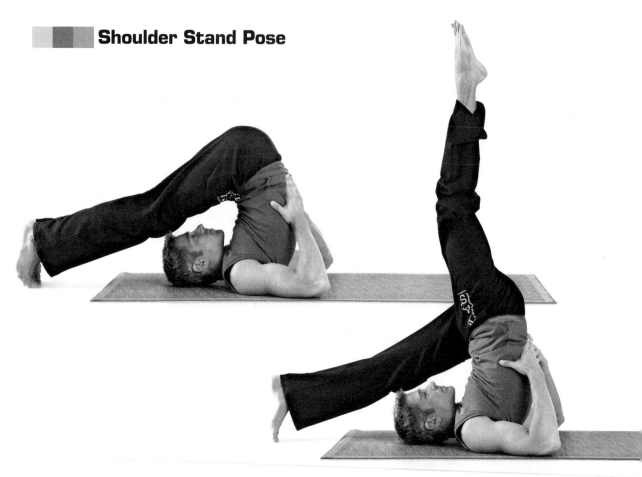

Benefits Shoulder Stand is what they call in yoga an "inversion"; you might hear a yoga instructor say, "We are going into our inversion poses." That basically means you are going upside down. You might hear your teacher talk about the "anti-aging" benefits of this pose. The practical application is that you are reversing gravity; gravity pulls you down, causing wrinkles. Shoulder Stand reverses that aging effect or at least tries to reverse it. I'm not going to promise you that you will look 10 years younger in a week, but it can't hurt to try to reverse gravity's effects. The main benefit is that this pose provides a great stretch for your neck and upper back.

How do you get into this pose?

- Lie on the floor on your back.
- Bring your arms alongside your body with your palms down.
- Bring your legs in the air, toward the ceiling.
- Press into your hands to lift your legs over your head, coming to Plow pose.
- Clasp your hands together and try to roll your shoulder blades toward each other.
- Bring your hands to your lower back for support; make sure your fingers are spread wide.

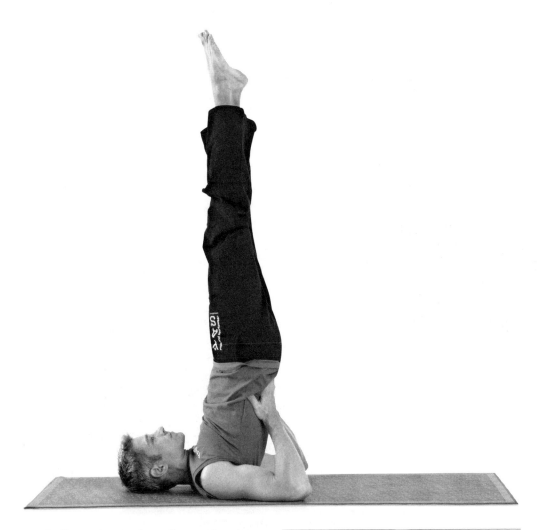

- Lift your legs to the ceiling one leg at a time. Take your time.
- Try to get as straight as possible, by walking your hands closer to your shoulders.
- Hold for 1 to 3 minutes.

Modify the Pose Put your feet up against a wall and lift your hips by pressing your feet into the wall.

Level of Difficulty Shoulder Stand is a more advanced pose. I would give it a solid 8.

QUICK-FIX TIPS Keep your weight on your triceps, not your neck. Use a blanket under your neck for support. You don't have to do Shoulder Stand to get the "anti-aging" benefits of an inversion—you can do a simple Legs Up the Wall pose or a Standing Forward Bend pose.

Knees to Ears Pose (aka Deaf Man's Pose)

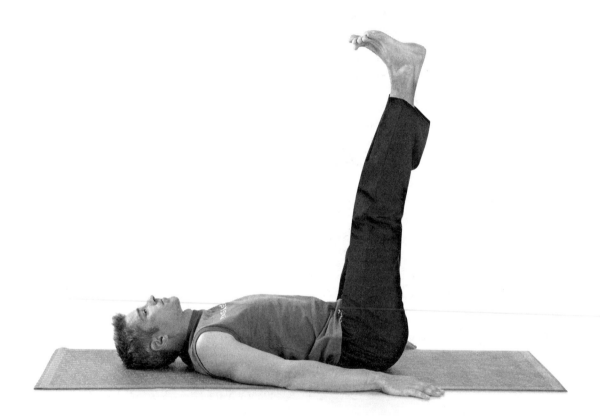

Benefits This pose is a great stretch for your neck, but doing the full pose takes a lot of flexibility. Once you are in the pose you will see why it's called Deaf Man's pose. After you master the pose it actually has a calming effect on your body.

How do you get into this pose?

■ From Plow, drop your knees around your ears.

■ Let your knees come to or toward the floor.

■ Hold for 30 seconds.

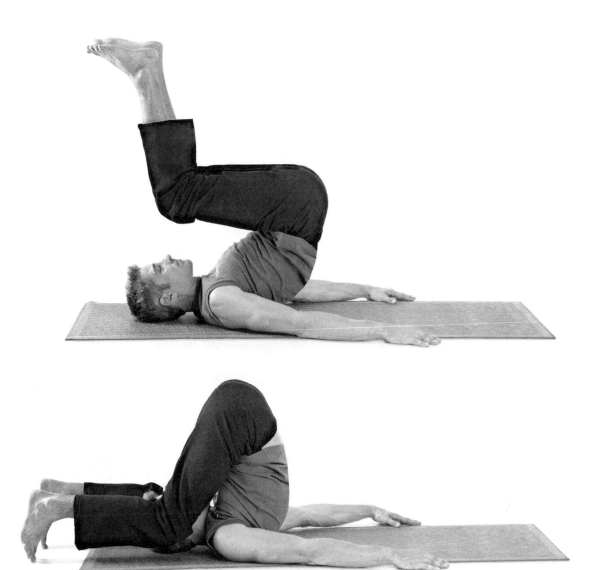

Modify the Pose Don't drop your knees down as far; instead, rest them on your forehead.

Level of Difficulty This pose can be an intense pose. I would rate it a 9.

QUICK-FIX TIP You can wrap your arms around the back of your thighs to intensify the pose.

Fish Pose

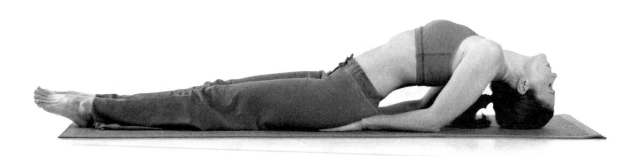

Benefits This pose is great for flexion of your neck because it decreases the angle between the head and the shoulders. It's a "counterpose" to sitting at your computer all day. That may be why you might find this pose hard, even though it seems like such a simple pose. Fish pose is a "traditional" counterpose to Shoulder Stand. This means that you may find yourself doing Fish pose after Shoulder Stand if you do yoga at your gym or at a yoga studio. Fish pose helps with backache and is said to help with fatigue and anxiety. In fact, this is one of those poses that a lot of yoga Web sites say cures everything from depression to menopause. From a practical standpoint, you can understand why Fish pose may help you with anxiety or depression. It opens up your neck and shoulders, which are areas in the body that hold a lot of stress. When you get depressed, your shoulders slump forward and you usually keep your head down. Fish pose stretches and strengthens the muscles in the back of your neck. It also helps with posture. Fish pose, like Bridge, is a backbend—it opens up the front of your body while strengthening the back of your body. This helps relieve stress and tension in the middle and upper part of your back.

QUICK-FIX TIP If you feel any discomfort in your neck, just lower your chest toward the floor so there isn't such a big arch in your back. Try not to scrunch your neck.

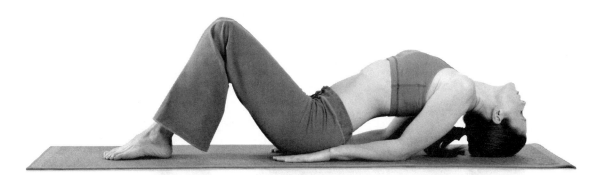

How do you get into this pose?

- Start lying down on your back, on the floor.
- Bring your hands, palms down, under your butt.
- Lean on and bend your elbows by pressing them into the floor.
- Lift your chest to the ceiling so your back is arched.
- Bring your elbows toward each other, as you did in Bridge and Shoulder Stand.
- Drop your head back, toward the floor behind you.

- Keep your legs straight and on the floor.
- Point your toes.
- Hold for 30 seconds.
- Release your arms and let your back roll down to the floor.

Modify the Pose Don't drop your head back. Bend your knees.

Level of Difficulty This pose is pretty easy, so I would rate it a 5.

"Yoga for Your Neck" Workout Routine: 10 Minutes

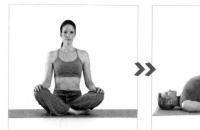

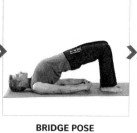

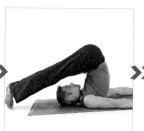

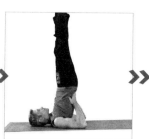

| **BREATH WORK** | **BRIDGE POSE** | **PLOW POSE** | **SHOULDER STAND POSE** |

Sit up tall in an easy cross-legged position and close your eyes. Take a minute to center your body and focus on your neck. Take a deep breath in through your nose and exhale it through your mouth. We're going to do this two more times. Each time, try to hold your breath for a few moments before you exhale.

Bring your knees together and roll down onto the floor; make sure you are on a padded surface, especially under your neck. We are going to do Bridge pose, so let your feet fall to the floor with your knees bent, bringing your feet about hip-distance apart. Reach down with your fingertips and see if you can feel your heels. If you can't, then move your heels a little closer to your body. Take a deep breath in, and on your exhale press into your feet to lift your hips up to the ceiling. Try to keep your thighs parallel—don't let your knees splay out. Once your hips are up, try to bring your arms underneath you and clasp your hands together. Try to roll your shoulder blades toward each other. Bring your chest toward your chin and your hips to the ceiling. Hold this for 45 seconds to 1 minute. You are opening the front of your body and strengthening your lower back. Release your arms and then slowly roll down to the floor. Repeat this two more times and then hug your knees into your chest and rock side to side.

From here we are going to do Plow pose. Now, if you have never done this pose before or if you have any neck issues, I would suggest just putting your legs up the wall. That pose is actually called Legs Up the Wall. Bring your legs straight up in the air toward the ceiling, bring your arms by your sides with your palms down, and take a deep breath in. On your exhale, press into your palms to lift your legs over your head. If you find your feet are not hitting the ground, then I want you to bring your hands to your lower back. If your feet are hitting the ground, you might want to try to do what you just did in Bridge pose—clasp your hands together and then try to roll your shoulder blades toward each other. That way you are setting yourself up for your next pose, Shoulder Stand.

From Plow, bring your hands to your lower back if they aren't already there. You want to make sure your lower back is supported first, and then bring your legs up to the ceiling one leg at a time. Take your time; in yoga, form is more important than speed. When you have both legs up in the air, toes pointed to the ceiling, see if you can bring your hands a little closer to your shoulders. Your weight should be on your triceps, not your neck. I want you to hold this pose for 1 to 3 minutes. Remember, this is your "anti-aging pose"—to really get the benefits of reversing gravity, you need to stay upside down for awhile. From here, just lower your legs over your head again, as you did in Plow pose.

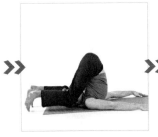

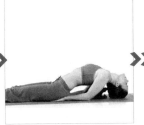

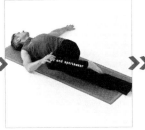

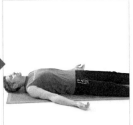

KNEES TO EARS POSE

FISH POSE

EASY SPINAL TWIST

CORPSE POSE

From Shoulder Stand, drop your legs over your head and, if you can, let your knees fall toward your ears. Hold this for 30 to 45 seconds; take a deep breath in, and on your exhale slowly let your whole body roll down onto the mat.

Once you are flat on the floor, we are going to do Fish pose. Bring your hands under your butt, with your palms down, press into your elbows to lift your chest up to the ceiling, and then let your head fall back, releasing any tension in your neck. This pose is a counterpose to Shoulder Stand, so you are stretching your neck forward in Shoulder Stand and then back with Fish pose. Release your arms and let your upper body come down flat on the floor. From here, hug your knees into your chest and rock side to side.

Bring your left knee into your chest and your right leg straight on the floor. Bring your left knee across your body while keeping your shoulder blades on the floor. Look over your left shoulder to complete this twist. Hold for 20 to 30 seconds, then hug both knees into your chest. Switch sides. Right knee comes into your chest, and left leg goes straight. Bring the right knee across your body and look over your right shoulder to complete the twist on the right side. Take a second to notice the difference from one side to the other. Hold for 20 to 30 seconds, then bring both knees into your chest.

I know most people want to skip this pose. But this pose allows your body to adjust to what you just did. It lets all the benefits of your "Yoga for the Neck" workout routine sink into your body. If you don't do Corpse pose, it's like having a massage, then hopping off the table and running off to work. The body needs a little time to readjust to get the most benefits from what you just did. So roll down onto the floor and then just let everything go. Bring your hands out by your sides, with your palms up. Close your eyes (if you have a towel close by, you may want to put the towel over your eyes). Take a deep breath in through your nose and let it out through your mouth. Do that two more times. Stay here for about 2 minutes to get the maximum benefits. After you are completely relaxed, take a deep breath in through your nose and just "sigh" it out. Then bend your knees, roll onto your right side for a few seconds, and push yourself up to a comfortable, easy, cross-legged position like the one we started with. Bring your hands together in front of your chest, take a deep breath in, and on your exhale bow forward. Take a second to appreciate the fact that you did something good for yourself today.

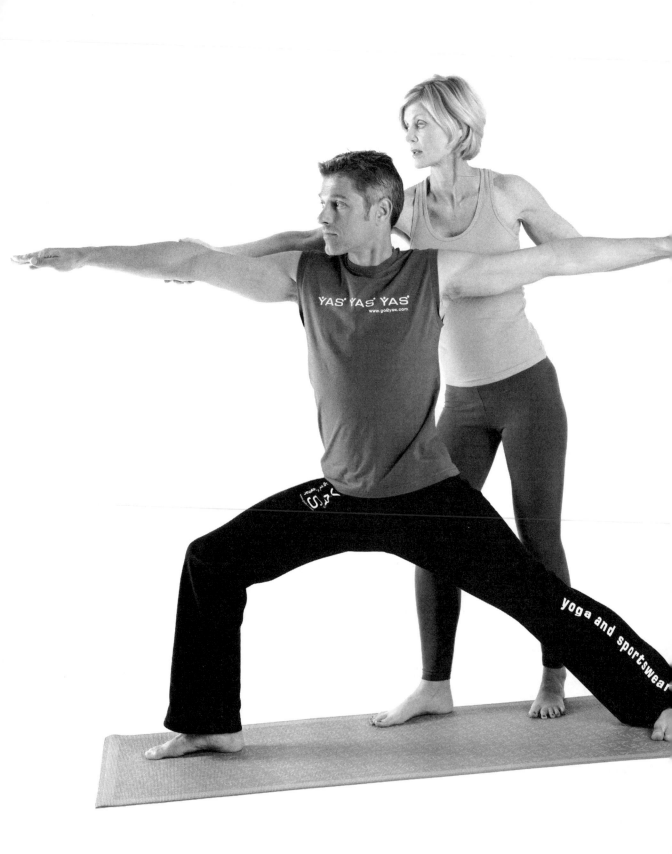

chapter 3

Shoulders

Does Yoga Make You Taller?

Over the years I have had so many students ask me, "Does yoga make you taller?" (To be honest, I would say that it is the *second* most common remark I get from guys who start taking my class. The first most common comment I get from them is, "Yoga is a lot harder than I thought it would be!") One of my students, who is a professional rugby player, asked me about yoga making him taller. He was very excited about being taller, even though he was already 6'5". In a way it does make you taller because it makes you stand up straighter. Your shoulders play an important role here because yoga causes them to roll back instead of forward, which gives you the appearance of being taller. Yoga helps your shoulders in many ways. The poses not only make them look better by toning them but also make them stronger and more flexible by stretching the muscle around them. All this will improve their range of motion.

Shoulder health is important to athletes who participate in all types of sports, including swimming, surfing, tennis, baseball, and basketball. I am personally very familiar with the muscles around the shoulders because I have spent many years rehabbing two broken collarbones, one from a biking accident and one from being thrown from my horse. Maybe someday I'll perfect the "tuck and roll." Having had a broken collarbone has prevented me from doing poses such as Wheel; I have to modify Wheel by doing Bridge instead. Remember, it doesn't make you less of a "yogi" if you have to modify a pose because of an injury. In fact, it makes you someone who is aware of your body's specific problem areas.

Shoulders, unfortunately, like the rest of our bodies, get really tight as we age; I've seen many students over the years who can't even raise their arms over their heads in poses such as Warrior 1 (see Chapter 11). Often this is caused by "frozen shoulder," which affects the shoulder joint (where the humerus bone fits into the socket of the shoulder). The ligaments and the surrounding capsule of the shoulder become inflamed, causing stiffness and a limited range of motion. This also happens after an injury to the shoulder. Fascia or scar tissue grows around the injury to protect it and stop it from moving. Once the injury is healed, however, the joint is still held in place by this surrounding fascia. So the goal in yoga is to loosen up the shoulder after an injury and allow it to move again.

For instance, with my own injury, I could not serve when I tried to play tennis. It was impossible to raise my arm over my head, and my serve looked like a cross-court forehand—not exactly what I was going for. Yoga helped loosen my shoulder to the point where I was back in the game. The pose I like the most to help in this situation is Downward-Facing Dog, which is why I included it in the "Yoga for Your Shoulders" workout routine.

If you are recovering from any type of shoulder injury, talk to your doctor first, and don't push yourself to the point where you are in pain. Remember that the "no pain, no gain" motto of most athletes doesn't work with yoga. One of the reasons yoga is so frustrating for athletes is that no matter how much you want to master a pose, you can't push yourself into it if your body is not ready. You should only go to a point where you feel a stretch; if you find yourself holding your breath or in pain in any pose, it's probably time to back off a bit.

How Do the Shoulders Work?

The causes of the more common injuries and pain of the shoulders are easier to understand if you have at least a little knowledge about their anatomy. The shoulder is pretty complex—it's made up of three bones, four muscles, and several tendons. Tendons attach the muscle to the bone. The bones of the shoulder are called the shoulder blade (scapula), the upper arm bone (the humerus), and the collarbone (the clavicle). The collarbone is an S-shaped bone that connects the shoulder to the breastplate, also called the sternum. The joint between the clavicle and the shoulder blade is called the acromion or A/C joint. The clavicle is designed to support the shoulder by aligning the shoulder with the rest of the chest.

The shoulder is the most mobile and flexible joint in the body and allows us to control where we can move our hands in order to use them. The very fine balance between mobility and stability in the shoulder gives us freedom of movement. The shoulder is a ball-and-socket joint, but it is very different from the hip joint, also a ball-and-socket joint. The hip joint has more natural stability than a shoulder joint because the ball of the hip

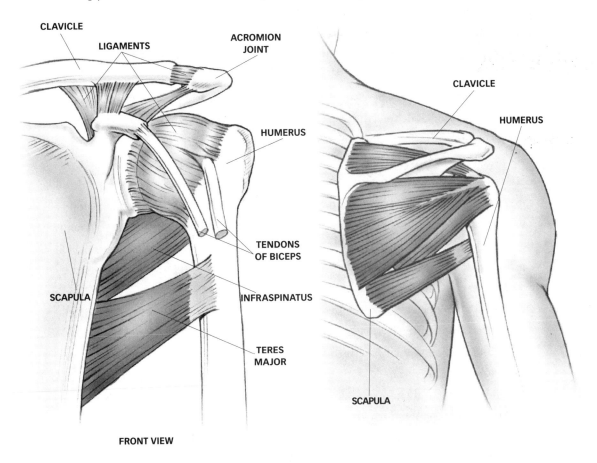

FRONT VIEW

is almost entirely surrounded by the socket of the pelvis. The shoulder, on the other hand, is controlled by a complicated arrangement of muscles, tendons, ligaments, and nerves, all in a balancing act. Injuries to the shoulder can upset the balance, causing a significant amount of pain and shoulder problems.

Common Shoulder Injuries

Rotator cuff tears: A torn rotator cuff is a common cause of pain and weakness in the shoulder. These tears have several different causes. We are going to take a look at why a torn rotator cuff happens and how yoga can help prevent it. The movement of your arm and shoulder is controlled by the four muscles that make up the rotator cuff. These muscles attach to the shoulder blade and then insert into the upper part of the humerus. They control the way in which the arm is rotated and how it is lifted up and down. At the end of each muscle is a tendon that attaches to the bone. Tears in these tendons are called rotator cuff tears.

Certain athletes, such as baseball players (particularly pitchers), and workers who often have their arms extended overhead, such as painters and dry wall installers, frequently develop tendinitis (inflammation in their shoulder joint). This inflammation causes pain and tenderness, and over time, the wear and tear on the rotator cuff can lead to a tear in one of the tendons. A direct blow to the shoulder, a fall onto an outstretched hand, or a dislocated shoulder joint can also result in a tear of one of the rotator cuff tendons. Another cause is related to the aging process—as we age, so does the rotator cuff. A process of natural wear and tear breaks down the strength and flexibility of the rotator cuff tendons, which can lead to a rupture of one of the tendons. Because yoga helps keep your shoulder strong and flexible, you can see why it would help prevent this type of injury.

Dislocated shoulder: A dislocated shoulder is relatively common, especially for people who play a lot of sports. So what is a dislocated shoulder? When the shoulder slips out of joint and the ball of the humerus is no longer resting in the socket of the scapula, the joint is said to be "dislocated." A dislocated shoulder is very painful. The muscles that move the shoulder tighten up and go into spasm after the shoulder has been dislocated, and they prevent the shoulder from going back into joint easily. A doctor usually has to move the shoulder in order to force it back into the joint. Ouch!

Shoulder fractures: The most frequent fracture of a shoulder bone is a broken collarbone. These injuries are very painful. I know from experience—I have broken my collarbone twice. I've been told having a broken collarbone is very common; I guess this is true, unless my doctor just told me this to make me feel less like a klutz! A broken collarbone usually occurs when someone falls onto an outstretched hand or onto the point of the shoulder (this is where the tuck and roll would come in handy). Most people know that they have broken a bone because they often hear the sound of the bone cracking and are in a lot of pain. Because the collarbone is very close to the skin, the swelling and the bruising are easily seen. These fractures usually heal very well on their own and do not require surgery.

Loose shoulder or shoulder instability: The capsule that surrounds the shoulder joint is a very strong ligament that helps to keep the shoulder in the joint and functioning normally. These injuries usually occur only when a lot of force has been applied to the shoulder or the arm—like being tackled in a football game. A dislocated shoulder occurs when the shoulder comes completely out of joint. This is a particularly big problem for "overhead athletes," such as baseball pitchers and tennis players, who depend on their shoulder to play their sport.

So what causes an unstable shoulder? A bad injury to the shoulder can cause the shoulder to become unstable by stretching or tearing the ligaments of the shoulder away from the bone. When the ligaments of the shoulder are pulled away from the bone, a Bankart lesion occurs. Shoulder instability can also be caused by a generalized looseness of the joints. Certain people are born with ligaments that are more loose than normal. These people are frequently very flexible and are often called "double-jointed." I have several students who are double-jointed, which in a way makes them too flexible.

POSES TO HELP YOUR SHOULDERS:

1. Reverse Prayer pose
2. Downward-Facing Dog pose
3. Upward-Facing Dog pose
4. Side-Angle pose with a twist
5. Inclined Plane pose
6. Seated Spinal Twist pose

Reverse Prayer Pose

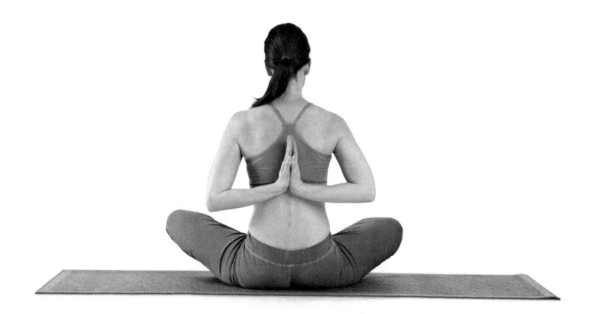

Benefits This pose loosens the shoulder joints by increasing the flexibility in your shoulders, chest, and upper back.

How do you get into this pose?

- Come to an easy cross-legged position on the floor.
- Bring your hands to your lower back with your palms facing each other.
- Try to bring your hands together in a prayer position.
- Bring your fingertips up your back as far as you can. Your goal should be to try to get your hands between your shoulder blades.
- Hold for 30 seconds to 1 minute.

Modify the Pose Instead of trying to bring your palms together behind your back, just clasp opposite elbows.

Level of Difficulty Well, I may be biased when it comes to this pose. Since I have broken my collarbone twice, this pose is brutal for me! I would still give it at least a 6.5.

Downward-Facing Dog Pose

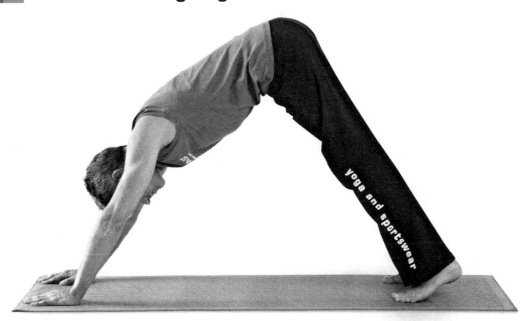

Benefits I'm sure most of you have heard of Downward-Facing Dog, right? It is one of the classic poses in yoga. Sometimes it's used as a "resting" pose in what is normally called a "flow" class, where you are moving from one pose to another. I love this pose—it's one of my favorites because I have very tight shoulders. If you have time to do only one shoulder pose, this is the one to do.

How do you get into this pose?

- Come down to the floor on your hands and knees.
- Bring your hands about shoulder-distance apart, palms flat on the floor.
- Bend your knees, engage your core muscles, and pull yourself back to what looks like an inverted V.
- Bring your feet about hip-distance apart.

QUICK-FIX TIP **To get more of a stretch in your shoulders and chest muscles, bend your knees and try to sink your chest toward your thighs.**

- Try to get your heels down and your butt up to the ceiling.
- Relax your neck.
- Hold for 45 seconds to 1 minute.

Modify the Pose Place your hands on the seat of a chair; this will help you get a good stretch in the shoulders.

Level of Difficulty This is normally an easy pose for most people, but for those of you with tight shoulders or hamstrings, it might not be as easy. So I would rate this pose a 6.5.

Upward-Facing Dog Pose

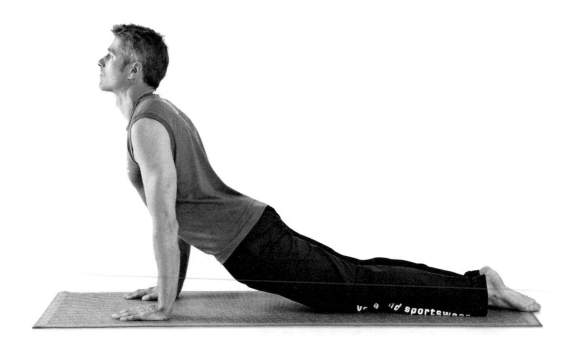

Benefits There are so many benefits to Upward-Facing Dog; opening up your chest muscles is just one of them. It improves your posture by opening not only the chest but also the shoulders. It also strengthens your arms, wrists, shoulders, and chest muscles.

How do you get into this pose?

- Lie down on your stomach.
- Bring your legs straight back behind you.

- Make sure the tops of your feet are on the floor.
- Bend your elbows and place your hands by your hips.
- Spread your fingertips wide apart.
- Press into your hands to straighten your arms.
- Lift your chest up and slightly back, if you can.
- Keep your thighs active.

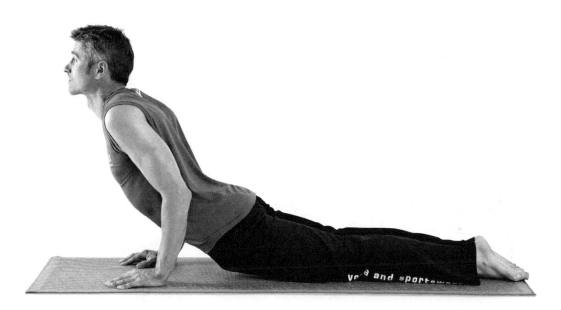

- Press into your hands and the tops of your feet; see if you can lift your thighs off the floor.
- Look straight ahead.
- Hold for 30 to 45 seconds.

Modify the Pose Bend your elbows to take the pressure off your lower back.

Level of Difficulty This is a hard one to rate. I find it very hard personally, and if you are new to yoga it might be hard for you, too. So I rate it a 7.

QUICK-FIX TIP To keep your shoulders away from your ears, drop your shoulder blades down your back and really open up your shoulders.

Side-Angle Pose with a Twist

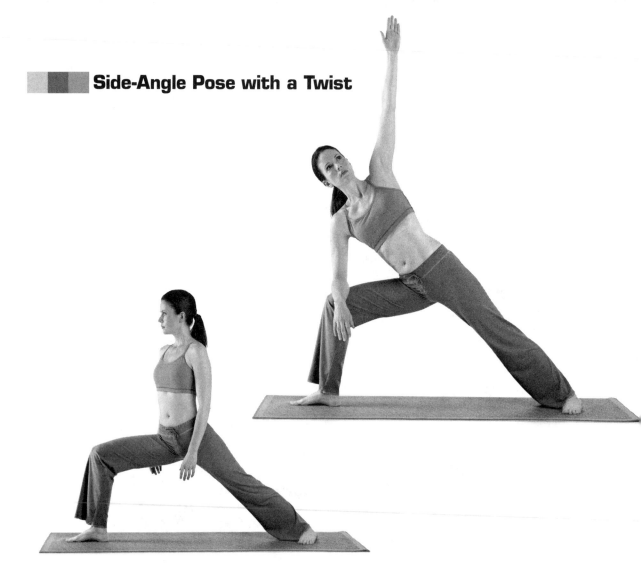

Benefits This pose opens the front of your body and works your lower body, but when you add the wrapping modification it becomes a shoulder opener as well.

How do you get into this pose?

■ Start standing; bring your left foot back about 3 to 4 feet, depending on your height and flexibility.

■ Bend your right knee until your thigh is level with the floor; if that's too much, then don't go down as far.

■ Your back heel should be flat on the ground at a 45-degree angle so that your heel is back and your toes are pointed slightly forward.

■ Bring your right hand to the inside of your knee. Alternately, rest your palm flat on the floor on the inside of your foot if you can do so without collapsing through your chest.

■ Bring your left arm straight up to the ceiling.

■ Let your left arm drop behind your back

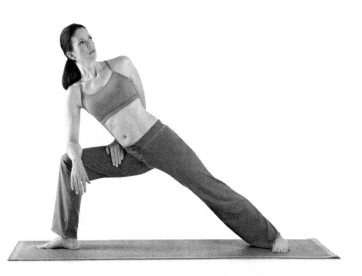

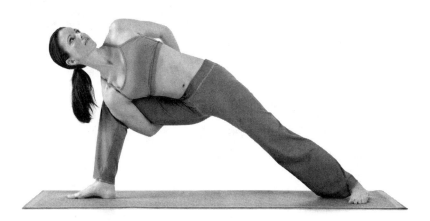

and then grab your thigh and rotate your chest to the ceiling.

■ You can look down to the side or up, depending on your flexibility; just go to your level.

■ Hold this for 45 seconds to 1 minute.

■ Switch sides. Stand up and shake out your legs.

■ Step your right foot back about 3 to 4 feet.

■ Bend your left knee this time.

■ Bring your left hand to the floor or to your knee depending on your flexibility.

Modify the Pose If you cannot bring your hand to the inside of your foot, or if you find your butt is sticking out, then bring your elbow to your knee until your hips open up a little more.

Level of Difficulty This is a hard pose, especially if your shoulders are tight. I would rate this pose a 7.5.

Inclined Plane Pose

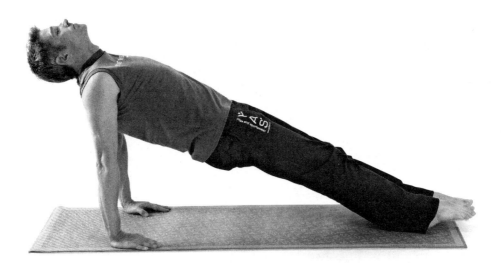

Benefits This pose builds strength in your shoulder, arms, chest area, wrists, and ankle joints. It also stretches your shoulders.

How do you get into this pose?

- Sit on the floor with your legs out in front of you.
- Put your hands behind your hips with your fingertips facing toward you.
- Press into your hands to raise your hips and chest toward the ceiling.

QUICK-FIX TIP Try not to crunch your neck; slowly let your head fall back.

- Keep your legs and arms straight.
- Drop your head back to stretch your neck.
- Hold for 30 seconds to 1 minute.
- Release your body to the floor, coming back to a sitting position.
- Repeat two more times.

Modify the Pose Only lift your hips as high as you can. You might not be perfectly flat, but you are still opening your shoulders.

Level of Difficulty Inclined Plane pose can be a hard pose if you have tight shoulders. I would rate it a 7.

Seated Spinal Twist Pose

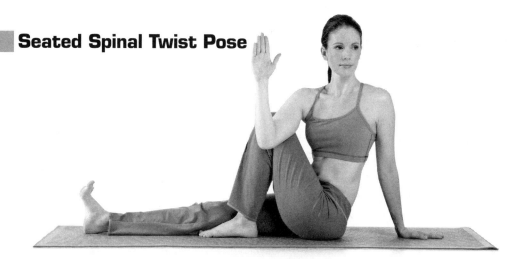

Benefits This pose releases tension in your shoulders, neck, and lower back. It relieves mild backache and hip pain by strengthening and stretching the muscles of the lower back. This pose helps with your lateral movement (that is, side-to-side or twisting movement), which is normally the first type of flexibility that is lost in your back. Remember, "no pain, no gain" does not apply to yoga. This should be a gentle stretch; twist just as far as is comfortable and focus on your upper back and shoulders, not your lower back.

How do you get into this pose?

- Sit on the floor with your legs out in front of you.
- Bend your left knee and bring it toward you.
- Keep your right leg on the floor.
- Lift your left leg over your right, and place your left foot on the floor next to your right knee.
- Keep your foot on the ground.
- Sitting with your spine straight, place your right elbow on the left side of your left knee.
- Bring your right hand behind you for support.
- Bend your left elbow and place your upper arm against the inside of your left

thigh, while at the same time twisting to look over your left shoulder.

- Press your left arm and knee against each other.
- Lift your torso and twist to the right. This is where you need to be careful not to twist too far.
- Keep your shoulders parallel and squared to the floor.
- Look over your right shoulder.
- Hold for 30 seconds to 1 minute.
- Repeat on the right side.

Modify the Pose Try to keep your back flat, but if you can't then sit up on a blanket.

Level of Difficulty This is a fairly easy pose; if your back isn't flexible, though, it may be a little challenging, so I would rate this pose a 5.5.

QUICK-FIX TIP Keep the straight leg on the ground; don't let your butt come off the floor. Remember to breathe—we have a tendency to hold our breath when we do twisting poses. Don't overtwist your neck; the focus of this pose is your shoulders.

"Yoga for Your Shoulders" Workout Routine: 10 Minutes

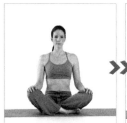 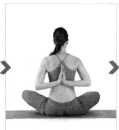 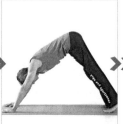 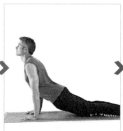 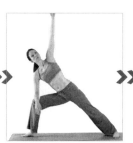

BREATH WORK

Come down to the floor—on your mat, if you have one. Sit in an easy cross-legged position, sit up tall, and close your eyes. We are going to take a minute to center your body and get you focused on your shoulders. Take a deep breath in through your nose and exhale it through your mouth. We're going to do this two more times; each time, try to hold your breath for a few moments before you exhale.

REVERSE PRAYER POSE

Stay seated in an easy cross-legged position on the floor, and switch legs. The leg behind now goes in front. Bring your hands to your lower back with your palms pressed together in a prayer position. Bring your fingertips up your back as far as you can. Hold for 30 seconds to 1 minute.

DOWNWARD-FACING DOG POSE

Come down to the floor on your hands and knees. Bring your hands about shoulder-distance apart, palms flat on the floor. Bend your knees, engage your core muscles, and pull yourself back to what looks like an inverted V. Bring your feet about hip-distance apart. Try to get your heels down and your butt up to the ceiling. Relax your neck. Hold for 45 seconds to 1 minute. You can bend your knees and sink your chest closer to your thighs to intensify this pose. This is one of my favorite poses for the shoulders.

UPWARD-FACING DOG POSE

From Downward-Facing Dog pose, drop down to your knees and lie down on your stomach. Bring your legs straight back behind you. Make sure the tops of your feet are on the floor. Bend your elbows and place your hands by your hips. Spread your fingertips wide apart. Press into your hands to straighten your arms. Lift your chest up and slightly back, bringing your shoulder blades together. Keep your thighs active by pressing the tops of your feet into the floor; see if you can lift your thighs off the floor. Look straight ahead. Hold for 30 to 45 seconds.

SIDE-ANGLE POSE WITH A TWIST

Push yourself back to Downward-Facing Dog. Let your right foot float to the ceiling and then swing it between your hands. Drop your back foot. Then come up to Warrior 1 position (see Chapter 11, Legs) for the benefits of the Warrior 1 pose. Bend your right knee until your thigh is level with the floor. If that's too much, then don't go down as far. Your back heel should be flat on the ground at a 45-degree angle so that your heel is back and your toes are pointed slightly forward. Bring your right hand to the inside of your foot, with your palm flat if you can. Bring your left arm straight up to the ceiling. Drop your top arm behind you, grab your right thigh, and try to twist toward the ceiling. Hold for 45 seconds to 1 minute. Switch sides. Step back to Downward-Facing Dog, this time letting your left leg float to the ceiling. Swing your foot between your hands and come up. Bend your left knee this time. Bring your left hand to the floor or to your knee, depending on your flexibility. Notice the difference between one side and the other.

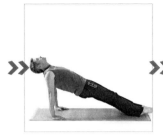

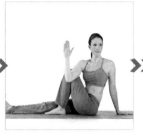

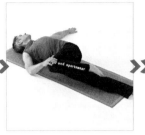

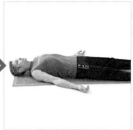

| **INCLINED PLANE POSE** | **SEATED SPINAL TWIST POSE** | **EASY SPINAL TWIST** | **CORPSE POSE** |

From Side-Angle pose, just go ahead and sit on the floor with your legs out in front of you. Put your hands behind your hips with your fingertips facing your hips. Bend your elbows. Press into your feet and your hands at the same time to lift your hips. Try to straighten your arms. Hold for 30 seconds to 1 minute. Repeat two more times.

From Inclined Plane pose, just drop your butt to the floor and bring both of your legs out in front of you. This pose involves twisting your back, so you should take particular care not to twist too far. We are focusing on your shoulders, not your lower back, but you get a nice stretch in your lower back as an added benefit. Bend your left knee, lift your left leg over your right, and place your left foot on the floor next to your right knee. Sitting with your spine straight, place your right elbow on the left side of your right knee. Bend your right arm so that your right fingertips are touching your left hip, while at the same time twisting to look over your left shoulder. This should be a gentle stretch; twist just as far as is comfortable. Hold for 45 seconds to 1 minute, release, and repeat on the opposite side.

From Seated Spinal Twist pose, just bring your knees together and roll down onto the floor. Bring your left knee into your chest and your right leg straight on the floor. Take a deep breath in, and on your exhale bring the bent knee across your body, keeping your shoulder blades on the floor. Look over your left shoulder to complete this twist. Bring both knees into your chest and then switch sides; the right knee comes into your chest, and left leg goes straight. Bring your knee across your body and hold for 45 seconds to 1 minute. Release and bring both knees into your chest. Then just let everything go down to the mat.

Lying flat on the floor, bring your arms out by your sides with your palms up; we are going to end this workout like we started it, with a little breath work, except you are going to be lying down instead of sitting up. Close your eyes, try to let your whole body relax, notice whether there is any tightness in your body, and relax that area. I want you to take a deep breath in, and bring the breath all the way through your body and exhale all the breath out. Do this two more times, focusing on relaxing your body. Stay here for about 2 minutes to get the maximum benefits. Bend your knees, roll onto your right side for a few seconds, then push yourself up to a comfortable, easy, cross-legged position like we started with. Bring your hands together in front of your chest, take a deep breath in, and on your exhale bow forward. Take a second to appreciate the fact that you did something good for yourself today. Your shoulders will thank you!

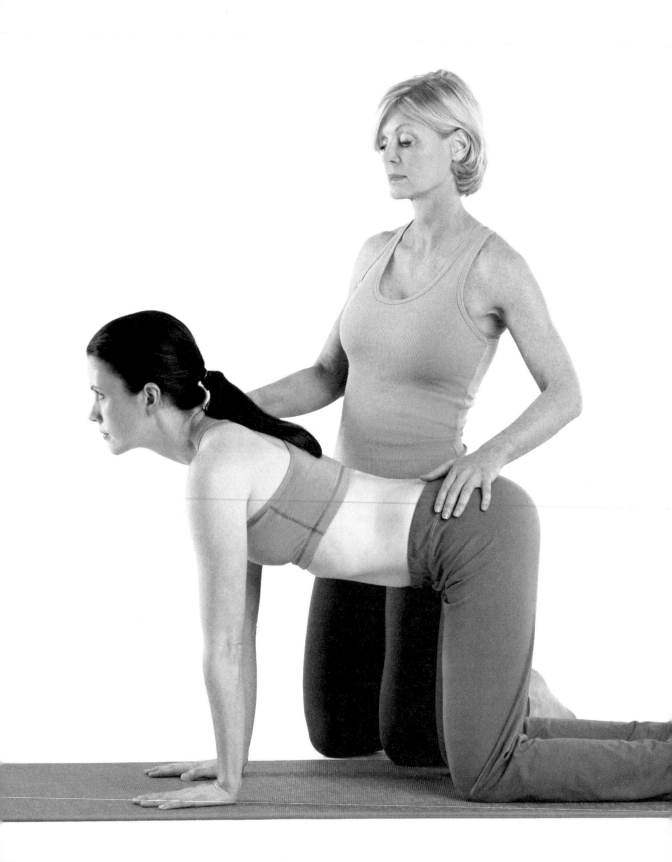

chapter 4

Upper Back

Where Are My Wings?

Your upper back, shoulders, neck, and chest are all intertwined with muscles, tendons, and ligaments, so the yoga poses that work on one of these areas will of course work on all the others, too. Bonus! The poses I have laid out here for your upper back workout routine are easier than the poses in some of the other chapters. The upper back doesn't have a lot of mobility, as you will see in the following discussion of how the upper back works. Because the movements are small and resistive, the poses are less challenging. The issues we deal with in this area are tightness from being at our computers all day or just bad posture in general. As we have already learned in the shoulder chapter, yoga is a great way to work on your posture. The best way to prevent upper back pain is to strengthen all your back and abdominal muscles, which protect your upper back. As with the rest of this book, if you have any upper back pain, make sure you ask your doctor before you do the "yoga for your upper back" workout routine.

How Does the Upper Back Work?

The upper back is called the thoracic spine, and it's composed of the middle 12 vertebrae of the back. Doctors often refer to these vertebrae as T1 to T12. The large bump on the lower part of the neck is the seventh cervical vertebra, called C7. The lowest vertebra of the thoracic spine, T12, connects below the bottom of the rib cage to the first vertebra of the lumbar spine, called L1. The main section of each thoracic vertebra from T1 to T12 is formed by a round block of bone called the vertebral body. Each vertebra increases

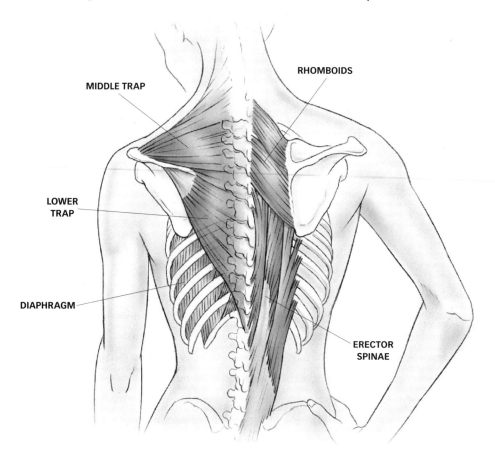

MIDDLE TRAP

RHOMBOIDS

LOWER
TRAP

DIAPHRAGM

ERECTOR
SPINAE

slightly in size from the neck down. The increased size helps balance and support the larger muscles, such as the extensor, flexor, and oblique muscles, that connect to the lower parts of the spine. Basically, it runs from the base of the neck to the bottom of the rib cage. Familiarizing yourself with the main parts of the thoracic spine and how they work can help you see how yoga can help your upper back.

The thoracic spine is very different from the cervical spine—the neck and the lumbar spine (the lower back)—because the neck and the lower back are designed to "move" to provide mobility in the spine. The thoracic spine is designed to be really strong and stable, meaning there isn't much movement in this area. One of the functions of the upper back area, and the reason it's meant to be strong, is that it protects our "vital organs," the ones we need to live (like the heart and lungs). The muscles of the upper back are arranged in layers. The ones closest to the skin's surface run from the back of the vertebrae to the shoulder blades. Others wrap around the rib cage and connect to the shoulders. Strap-shaped muscles called erector spinae make up the middle layer of muscles. These muscles run up and down over the lower ribs and the rib cage and cross to the lower back. The deepest layer of muscles attaches along the back of the spinal bones, connecting the vertebrae and each rib.

The poses for the upper back are limited because it has a limited range of motion. Generally speaking, this means there is little risk for injury in the upper back. Most sports injuries involve the lower back or neck; because the upper back is immobile, it's less likely to be injured during participation in sports.

Common Injuries of Your Upper Back

Because the upper back is shaped for support and protection, most serious joint conditions affecting the neck or lower back, such as spinal stenosis, disk injuries, and degeneration, are far less common in this area. In fact, this thoracic area often has to compensate for problems located in the lower back, neck, and shoulders. Injury to the joints of the upper back can be from intense twisting movements, especially if you are using weights and move awkwardly from the shoulders (I'm sure you have seen guys at the gym using weights they can barely lift). Any sport that involves a throwing action or repetitive practice of a certain stroke in racquet sports can result in an injury to this area. Viruses or extreme coughing or other internal problems can also cause upper back problems. When you have upper back pain, it is often difficult to relate it to the injury—you can have a lot of pain for a slight injury and very little pain for a more serious injury. You may feel a slight strain in your upper back and shoulder, or you may feel upper back and neck pain. This may occur only when you are playing sports, which suggests an injury that has come on gradually from the particular movement of that sport. Obviously, serious upper back injuries are usually easier to diagnose because there is typically severe pain and immobility; with such injuries, even breathing can cause pain.

Thoracic intervertebral joint sprain: The intervertebral joint joins the levels of the spine together. Injury to this joint is usually due to a forced movement of the thoracic spine forward or backward. Pain may radiate around the chest wall to the front of the chest. Pain is increased with forward or backward movement of the spine.

Thoracic muscle rupture: This injury is common in many sports, such as throwing sports, football, basketball, and boxing. It commonly occurs when lifting heavy objects. Symptoms include deep sharp pain when bending forward and backward, as well as rotating, side-to-side movement. There will also be localized tenderness around the area of injury in the back.

Rib fracture: This injury is very common in contact sports, such as football and rugby. It most commonly results from a blow to the ribs. Symptoms are very sharp pain to the touch, as well as discomfort and clicking with a deep breath, coughing, or sneezing. This injury commonly remains painful for a long time because of constant movement of the chest wall with breathing.

Scoliosis (curvature of the spine): This sideways spinal curvature causes the spine to be S-shaped. Symptoms of scoliosis are not always apparent. They include complications due to muscle weakness and joint looseness on one side and muscle tightness and spasm with joint tightness on the other side. The symptoms vary but tend to be aggravated by prolonged sitting or standing.

POSES TO HELP YOUR UPPER BACK:

1. Eagle pose: arms only

2. Reverse Prayer pose

3. Cobra pose

4. Cat-Cow pose

5. Thread the Needle pose

Eagle Pose: Arms Only

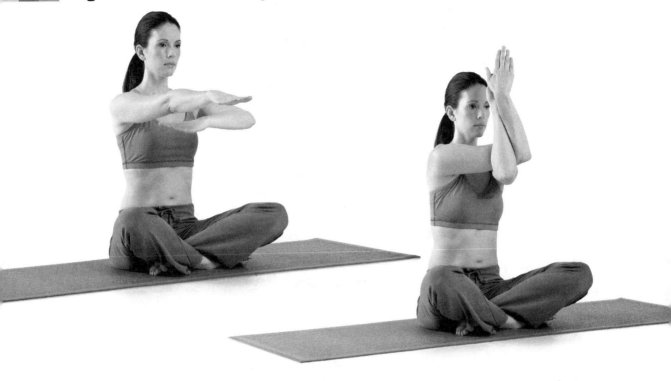

Benefits This pose opens the upper back by stretching your trapezius and rhomboid muscles. You can do this pose at your desk at work. It may look strange, but it feels great! The full pose, done standing, can be more difficult, so if you feel like challenging yourself you can try full Eagle (see Chapter 13, Feet and Ankles).

How do you get into this pose?

- Sit down on the floor in an easy cross-legged position.
- Bring your right arm straight out in front of you, as if you were going to shake someone's hand.
- Bring your left arm under the right arm.
- Bend both arms and try to bring your palms together in front of your face.

- Hold for 30 seconds to 1 minute.
- Switch sides.

Modify the Pose To intensify this pose, bring your elbows up.

Level of Difficulty 5.5. This could be higher for you, depending on the flexibility of your shoulders and upper back.

QUICK-FIX TIP **If you are having a hard time bringing your hands together, use a strap or a towel until your upper back loosens up.**

Reverse Prayer Pose

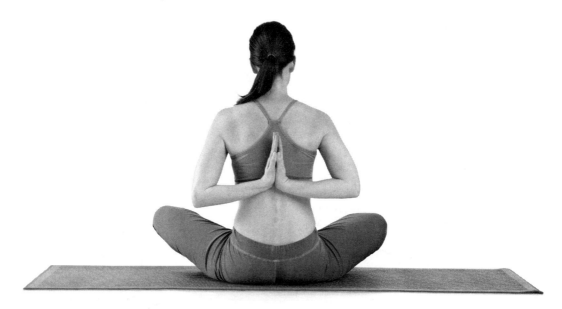

Benefits This pose helps with the flexibility of your shoulders and your upper back. It also develops arm strength. This is another pose that you can easily adapt to do at your desk.

How do you get into this pose?

- Come to an easy cross-legged position on the floor.
- Bring your hands to your lower back with your palms facing each other.
- Try to bring your hands together in a prayer position.
- Bring your fingertips up your back as far as you can. Your goal should be to try to get your hands between your shoulder blades.
- Hold for 30 seconds to 1 minute.

Modify the Pose Instead of trying to bring your palms together behind your back, just clasp opposite elbows.

Level of Difficulty Well, I may be biased when it comes to this pose. Since I have broken my collarbone twice, this pose is brutal for me! I would still give it at least a 6.5.

QUICK-FIX TIP **Keep your shoulders squared while you do this pose and remember to breathe.**

Cobra Pose

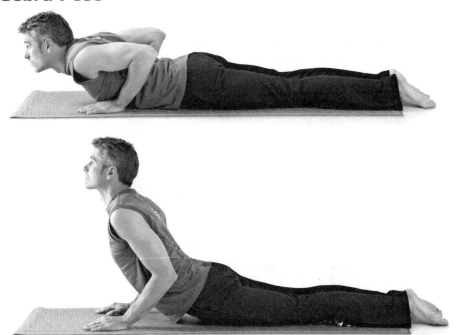

Benefits This pose stretches the spine and strengthens the upper back. It increases the mobility of your spine, especially your upper back and the middle of your back. It also stretches and strengthens your neck, shoulders, and chest. It's hard to do any pose for the upper back that doesn't also help these areas, since they are all connected.

How do you get into this pose?

- Lie down on your stomach with your forehead on the ground.
- Keep your legs together, with your feet and toes pointed straight back.
- Bring your hands flat on the ground under your shoulders, fingers spread wide.
- Keep your elbows in by your sides.
- Slowly raise your head and chest as high as they will go.
- Make sure your elbows stay bent.

- Look up; if you have any neck issues, then just look straight ahead.
- Keep your glutes tight to protect your lower back.
- Keep your head and chest up.
- Roll your shoulder blades down your back.
- Hold for 45 seconds to 1 minute.
- Repeat two times.

Modify the Pose Don't bring your chest up as high.

Level of Difficulty This is an easy pose for most people. It's a lot easier than Upward-Facing Dog, but I would still give it a 6.

QUICK-FIX TIP Bring your hands off the floor and see how high you can keep your chest up; this is as far as you should go to gently open your upper back.

Cat-Cow Pose

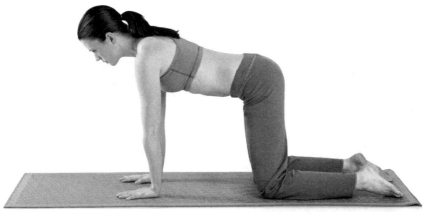

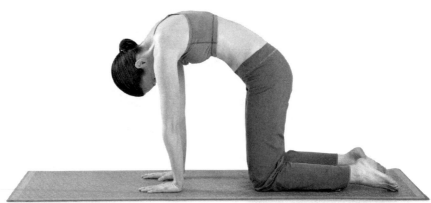

Benefits This pose stretches your upper back and adds flexibility to your lower back muscles.

How do you get into this pose?

- Start on your hands and knees.
- Bring your hands to about shoulder-distance apart.
- Bring your knees directly below your hips.
- Push into your hands to round your spine.
- Look toward your belly button.
- Let your head drop down, releasing your neck.

- Bring your head up.
- Let your lower back drop toward the floor.
- Do this 10 times.

Modify the Pose If you have lower back issues, then just do the Cat section of the pose instead of sinking your hips into the Cow part.

Level of Difficulty I would rate it a 4.5; this is a pretty easy pose.

QUICK-FIX TIP
Don't overextend your neck.

Thread the Needle Pose

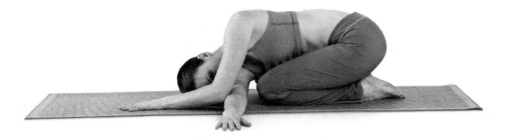

Benefits Thread the Needle pose stretches not only your upper back but also your shoulders, arms, and neck.

How do you get into this pose?

■ Come down to the floor on your hands and knees.

■ Balancing on your left hand, bring your right arm along the floor between your left hand and your left knee.

■ Your right shoulder and the right side of your face should be flat on the floor.

■ Bend the elbow of your left arm.

■ Hold for 30 seconds to 1 minute, depending on how this feels to you.

■ Release by pressing into your left palm.

■ Switch sides.

Modify the Pose To take this pose to the next level, bring your top arm to the ceiling, which will intensify the stretch in your upper back.

Level of Difficulty This is a pretty easy pose for most people, so I would rate it a 5.

QUICK-FIX TIP Since the side of your face will be planted on the floor, you will want to be on a mat or a padded surface when you do this pose.

"Yoga for Your Upper Back" Workout Routine: 8 Minutes

Because the upper back isn't really meant to move–and because most of the yoga poses that supposedly are for your upper back are actually for your shoulders, neck, and chest–we are only going to do poses that are fairly easy.

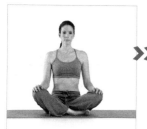 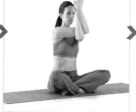 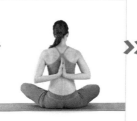 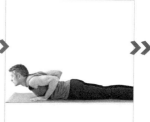

| BREATH WORK | HALF EAGLE POSE | REVERSE PRAYER POSE | COBRA POSE |

BREATH WORK

Come down to the floor—on your mat, if you have one. If you are doing this while you are at work, you can stay seated in your chair. If you are on the floor, situate yourself in an easy cross-legged position. Sit up tall and close your eyes. Take a minute to center your body and get focused on loosening your upper back. Take a deep breath in through your nose and exhale it through your mouth. Repeat this two more times. Each time try to hold your breath for a few moments before you exhale.

HALF EAGLE POSE

Stay seated, but switch legs. If your right leg is in front, switch to your left leg. Bring your right arm out in front of you as if you were about to shake someone's hand. Bring your left arm under your right and then bend both elbows to bring your hands in front of your face with your palms facing each other. Try to raise your elbows up; the higher you can bring your elbows up, the more of a stretch you will feel in your upper back. Hold for 45 seconds to 1 minute and release. Now switch sides so that your left arm comes out and your right arm goes underneath. Bend both elbows again and bring your hands in front of your face. See if you can get your elbows a little higher this time. Hold for 45 seconds to 1 minute.

REVERSE PRAYER POSE

Stay seated in an easy cross-legged position on the floor, and switch legs. The leg behind now goes in front. Bring your hands to your lower back with your palms pressed together in a prayer position. Bring your fingertips up your back as far as you can. Hold for 30 seconds to 1 minute.

COBRA POSE

Lie down on your stomach. Keep your legs together, with your upper arms at your sides and close to your body and your hands about mid-chest level. Take a deep breath in; on your exhale, slowly raise your head and chest as high as they will go. Look up or straight ahead, depending on the flexibility of your neck. Keep your buttock muscles tight to protect your lower back. Keep your head and chest up, and roll your shoulder blades down your back. Hold for 45 seconds to 1 minute. Repeat two more times. Push yourself back to Child's pose for a few seconds (see Chapter 9, Lower Back, for benefits of Child's pose).

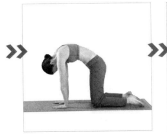 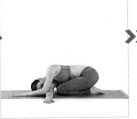 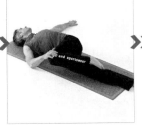 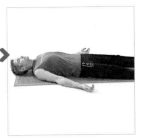

CAT-COW POSE

Come to all fours for Cat-Cow pose. Bring your hands about shoulder-distance apart and your knees about hip-distance apart. Keep your back flat for now. Take a deep breath in; on your exhale, push into your hands, drop your head, and round your back. Think of a cat when it gets all "puffed up." From here take a deep breath in; on your exhale, bring your head up and let your lower back sink down toward the floor. Repeat five to 10 times.

THREAD THE NEEDLE POSE

Stay on all fours and then bring your right arm under your left armpit. Balancing on your left hand, bring your right arm along the floor between your left hand and your left knee. Your right shoulder and the right side of your face should be flat on the floor. Bend the elbow of your left arm. Hold for 30 seconds to 1 minute, depending on how this feels to you. Release by pressing into your left palm. Repeat on the left side.

EASY SPINAL TWIST

Bring both knees into your chest and gently rock side to side. Then bring your left knee into your chest and stretch your right leg straight out on the floor. Take a deep breath in; on your exhale, bring the bent knee across your body, keeping your shoulder blades on the floor. Look over your left shoulder to complete your twist. Bring both knees into your chest and then switch sides—your right knee comes into your chest, and the left leg goes straight. Hold for 45 seconds to 1 minute, then release. Bring both knees into your chest. From here, we are going into our final pose.

CORPSE POSE

Take a deep breath in; on your exhale, let your whole body come to the floor. Place your arms out by your sides with your palms up. You are ending this workout like we started it, with a little breath work. Remember, don't skip this part. It helps the body adjust to what you just did. It allows the benefits of the routine to sink into your body before you run off to tackle the rest of the day. Close your eyes, and try to let your whole body relax. Take a deep breath in. Exhale, and repeat this two more times, focusing on relaxing your body. Stay here for about 2 minutes to get the maximum benefits. After you are completely relaxed, take a deep breath in through your nose and just "sigh" it out. Bend your knees and roll onto your right side for a few seconds. Then push yourself up to a comfortable cross-legged position like we started with. Take a second to appreciate the fact that you did something good for yourself today—your upper back will thank you!

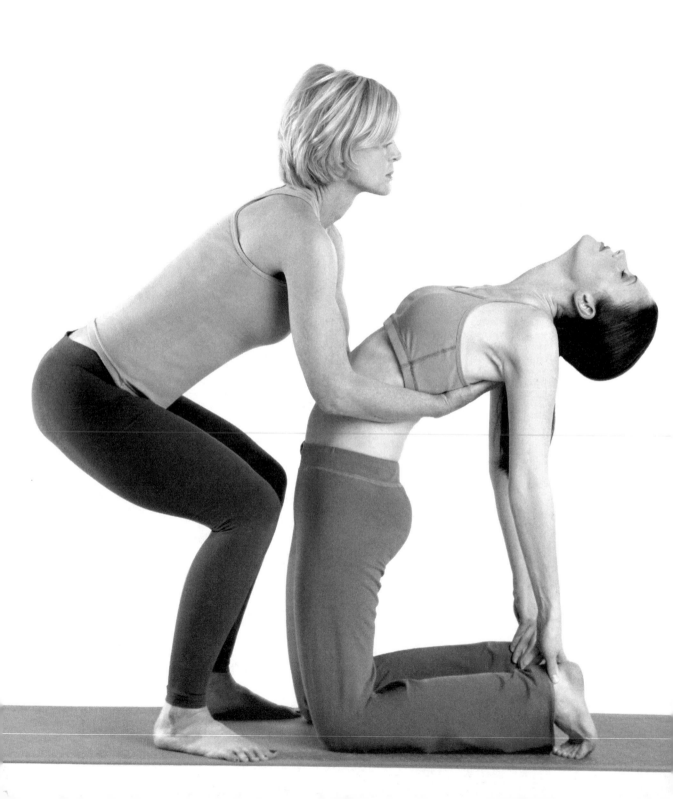

chapter 5

Chest

Puff It Up

When you think of your chest, what do you think—what visions come to mind? If you are a guy, you probably think of your "pecs," the pectoralis majors. If you're a woman, a whole other thing comes to mind. Well, the great thing about yoga is that, whether you are a male or a female, you will have a good-looking chest from doing it! That alone should make you want to give it a try.

The chest area is also where your heart is, both physically and emotionally. I start all my yoga classes with the question, "Does anyone have any injuries?" This is an important question so I can give students modifications for existing injuries. When I asked this question in one of my classes, a beautiful woman (and very famous actress) said,

"My heart is broken." The whole class in unison said, "Awww." I have to admit it threw me off for a second, for someone to be that open and vulnerable in front of a large group of people. I hope she wasn't acting! I did learn something from the reaction of the class—that everyone felt for her. Most of the women in the class instinctively put their hands over their hearts when she said it. The guys, on the other hand, well, their faces lit up, as they thought, "Wow, she's single?!" I suggested that she focus on her Camel pose.

There are poses in this section, such as Camel pose, that are referred to as "heart openers." Now, as you already know, I'm not a "woo woo" person, but in all my years of teaching and leading teacher trainings, I have seen people get very emotional after doing Camel. In one of my teacher trainings, I was working with a student who was having a trust issue with Camel pose. She was afraid that she couldn't reach her heels when she was going back into the pose. I told her just to trust that she could do the pose; when she did it, she had a total emotional release. If this happens to you while you are doing any of the poses, realize that it's okay.

Our bodies hold a lot of emotions; that's the whole theory behind Rolfing. If you haven't heard of Rolfing, it's similar to a deep massage, but it works on the connective tissue to release, realign, and balance the body. It helps get rid of pain and discomfort from many different causes, including back pain, repetitive motion injury, trauma, and aging. Rolfing is a great complement to your yoga practice. It's not the most pleasant experience you will ever have because it can be painful. If you are like me and have had a lot of trauma in your life, it may be worth looking into.

How Does the Chest Work?

When it comes to the chest in yoga, it's hard to separate it from your shoulders and upper back because they are all connected. But let's take a look at how the chest works. Your "pecs," which is what you think of as your chest, basically start at your breastbone (the center of your chest) and fan out to attach to your shoulder joints. The chest is made up of 12 ribs and the two layers of intercostal muscles. These small muscles are

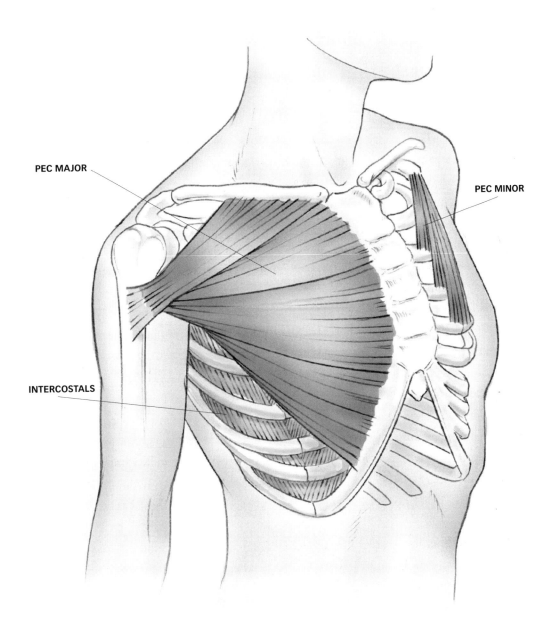

PEC MAJOR

PEC MINOR

INTERCOSTALS

called "intrinsic" muscles because they lie under the bigger muscle groups. The ribs start at the front of the body with the sternum (the breastbone). The sternum starts at the collarbone.

Common Injuries of the Chest

Many illnesses are associated with chest pain. Heart attack is chief among them. Heart disease is the leading cause of death in the United States, killing one in five people. But here is the good news: Between 1950 and 1999, the death rate from heart disease fell by almost 60% and is still falling, mostly because people are working out more. It is becoming clear that 80 to 90% of the people who develop coronary artery disease have at least one major controllable risk factor. Most of these risk factors can be eliminated or at least managed if you take steps to protect yourself, which means exercising. A yoga workout is a good way to help your heart.

When it comes to actual injury to the chest, you can injure the area indirectly as a result of forces transmitted through the chest or directly from trauma to the chest. The possible causes of chest pain in athletes can be divided into those arising from the ribs, the sternum, and the joints.

Stress fracture of the ribs: We have 24 ribs: 12 on each side. Stress fracture is most likely to occur in the first rib. Overhead athletes such as basketball or tennis players are typically at risk here because this area is often engaged in this type of activity or left vulnerable. If you have a stress fracture, you will feel pain around the shoulder or front of the neck. You may also feel tenderness at the top of the shoulder blade near your neck. Stress fractures to the other ribs are less common but are seen in such athletes as golfers and rowers.

Acute rib fractures: These are the result of direct injury. Fractures of the first and second ribs suggest a very significant transfer of energy and can be associated with underlying injuries. Now I have firsthand experience, unfortunately, with acute rib fractures. I know personally that you feel a sharp pain in the chest, which is aggravated by deep breathing or coughing.

POSES TO HELP YOUR CHEST:

1. Standing Forward Bend pose (arms overhead)

2. Humble Warrior pose

3. Twisted Chair pose

4. Camel pose

Standing Forward Bend Pose (Arms Overhead)

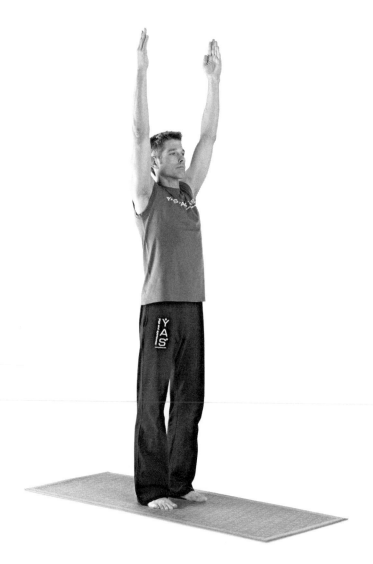

Benefits This pose opens up the chest and shoulders while strengthening your legs.

How do you get into this pose?

■ Come to a standing position with your feet about hip-distance apart and arms outstretched.

■ Bring your arms behind your back and clasp your hands together.

■ Hinge forward from your hips.

■ Bring your hands over your head.

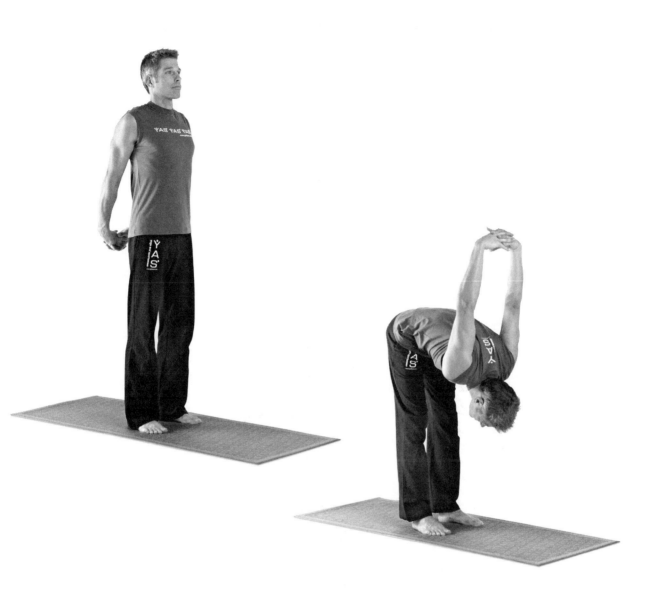

Modify the Pose If you cannot clasp your hands together, use a strap or a towel to bridge the gap.

Level of Difficulty This is a fairly easy pose, unless your chest is tight. I would give it a 6.

QUICK-FIX TIP You are working on your chest, so if you are feeling this in your hamstrings, just bend your knees to transfer the stretch to your chest.

Humble Warrior Pose

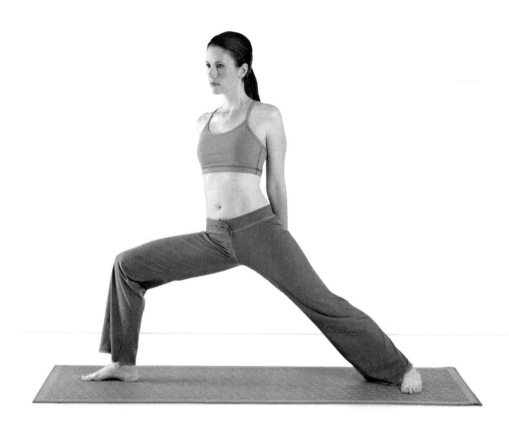

Benefits The arm part of this pose opens your chest and shoulders; the leg part you might recognize as a typical Warrior stance.

QUICK-FIX TIP **Don't let your knee buckle in or your butt stick out.**

How do you get into this pose?

■ Bring your legs about 3 to 4 feet apart.

■ Turn your right foot out and your left foot in as if you were going to do Warrior 1 (see Chapter 11).

■ Bend your right knee to a 90-degree angle.

■ Bring your arms behind you and clasp your hands together.

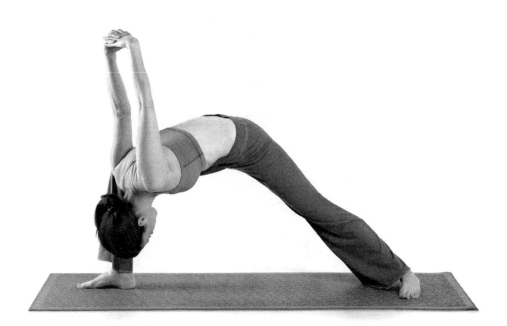

- Bend forward toward your front foot, and bring your arms over your head.
- Drop your head toward the floor.
- Hold for 45 seconds to 1 minute.
- Use your arms to pull you up so that you open your chest the whole way up.
- Release your arms.
- Switch sides.

Modify this Pose Don't drop your hands over your head; just focus on opening your chest area.

Level of Difficulty I would rate this pose a 6. As with all the other poses, this may be hard or easy for you depending on the flexibility of your shoulders and hips.

Twisted Chair Pose

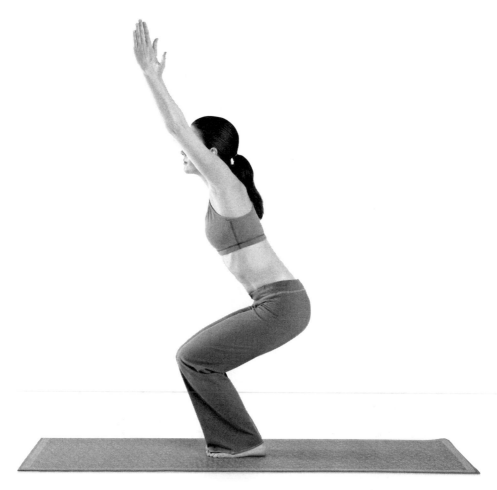

Benefits This pose is an advanced version of Chair (see Chapter 13, Feet and Ankles). This why we call it Twisted Chair or Chair with a Twist.

How do you get into this pose?

■ Stand up.

■ Bring your legs together, feet touching.

■ Sink down like you were about to sit on a chair.

■ Bring your hands together in front of your chest.

■ Bring your right elbow to your left knee.

■ Twist your chest to the ceiling.

■ Hold for 30 to 45 seconds.

■ Switch sides.

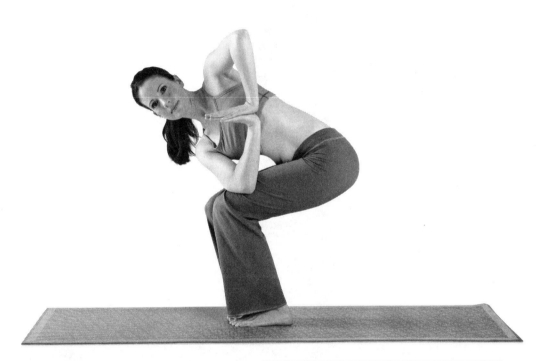

Modify the Pose You can make this pose more challenging by bringing your bottom hand to the floor and your top hand to the ceiling.

Level of Difficulty This pose is hard! It's an advanced version of Chair pose, so don't get frustrated if you can't hold this pose very long. I would rate this pose an 8.5.

QUICK-FIX TIP **Remember to breathe. Many people have a tendency to hold their breath in twisting poses.**

Camel Pose

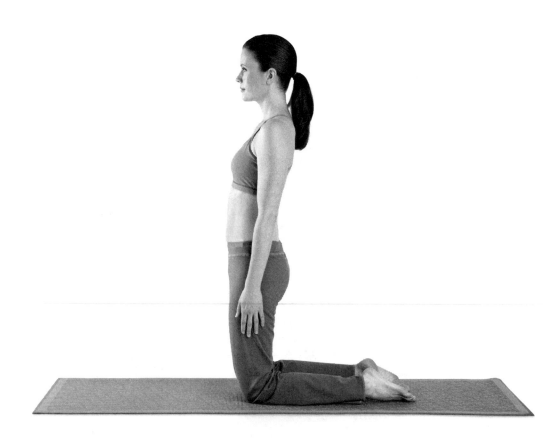

Benefits This pose stretches the whole front of your body and improves the flexibility of your spine. It also stretches your hip flexors, strengthens your back, and really helps your posture.

How do you get into this pose?

- Come down to the floor on your knees.
- Bring your legs hip-distance apart.

- Tuck your toes back.
- Bring your hands to your lower back.
- Let your head and chest fall back.
- Bring your hands to your heels. If you cannot reach your heels, then keep your hands on your lower back.
- Bring your hips forward.

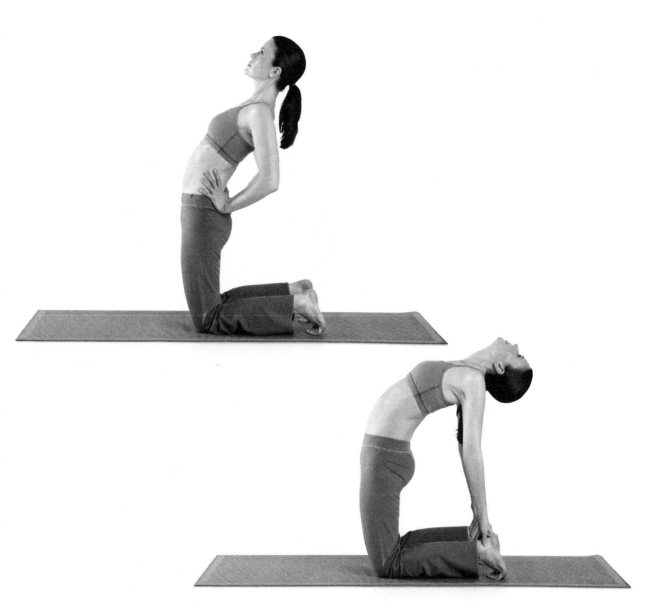

Modify the Pose If you have any neck issues, just keep your head up. If you cannot reach your heels, keep your hands on your lower back.

Level of Difficulty This pose is challenging, especially for those of us who sit at a computer all day. I would rate this pose a 7.5.

QUICK-FIX TIP **Make sure you are on a padded surface, especially if you have sensitive knees.**

"Yoga for Your Chest" Workout Routine: 8 Minutes

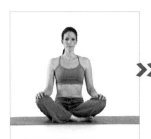

BREATH WORK

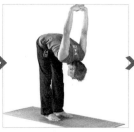

STANDING FORWARD BEND POSE (ARMS OVERHEAD)

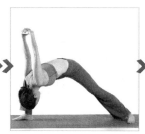

HUMBLE WARRIOR POSE

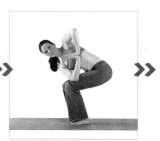

TWISTED CHAIR POSE

Come down to your mat. Sit in an easy cross-legged position with one leg in front of the other. Sit up tall and close your eyes. Take a minute to center your body and focus on your chest. Take a deep breath in through your nose and exhale it through your mouth. Repeat this two more times. Each time, try to hold your breath for a few moments before you exhale.

Come to a standing position. Bring your legs together with your arms behind you. Clasp your hands together, hinge at your waist, and bring your arms over your head.

Bring your legs about 3 to 4 feet apart. Turn your right foot out and your left foot in, as if you were going to do Warrior 1. Bend your right knee to a 90-degree angle. Bring your arms behind you and clasp your hands together. Bend forward toward your front foot, and bring your arms over your head. Drop your head toward the floor. Hold for 45 seconds to 1 minute. Use your arms to pull yourself up so that you open your chest the whole way up. Release your arms.

Remain standing and bring your legs together with your feet touching. Sink down as if you were about to sit on a chair. Bring your hands together in front of your chest. Bring your right elbow to your left knee. Twist your chest to the ceiling. Hold for 30 to 45 seconds. Switch sides.

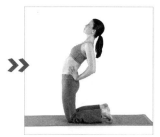

CAMEL POSE

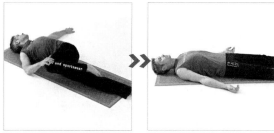

EASY SPINAL TWIST

CORPSE POSE

From Chair pose, come down to the floor on your knees. Bring your legs hip-distance apart. Tuck your toes back. Bring your hands to your lower back. Let your head and chest fall back. Bring your hands to your heels. If you cannot reach your heels, try to keep your hands on your lower back. Bring your hips forward. Imagine you are pushing the front of your thighs into the wall. This will help bring your hips forward.

To release your lower back from Camel, bring your left knee into your chest and let your right leg go straight on the floor. Take a deep breath in; on your next exhale, bring the bent knee across your body, keeping your shoulder blades on the floor. Look over your left shoulder to complete this twist. Bring both knees into your chest and then switch sides; the right knee comes into your chest, and the left leg goes straight. Hold for 45 seconds to 1 minute. Release and bring both knees into your chest. From here we are going into our final pose.

Bring your whole body to the floor. Hold your arms out by your sides with your palms up; we are going to end this workout like we started it, with a little breath work. Close your eyes, try to let your whole body relax, notice whether there is any tightness in your body, and relax that area. I want you to take a deep breath in, pretend that you are breathing from your feet, and bring the breath all the way through your body and exhale all the breath out. Repeat two more times. Stay here for about 2 minutes to get the maximum benefits. After you are completely relaxed, take a deep breath in through your nose and just "sigh" it out. Bend your knees, roll onto your right side for a few seconds, then push yourself up to a comfortable, easy cross-legged position like we started with. Bring your hands together in front of your chest, take a deep breath in, and on your exhale bow forward. Take a second to appreciate the fact that you did something good for yourself today!

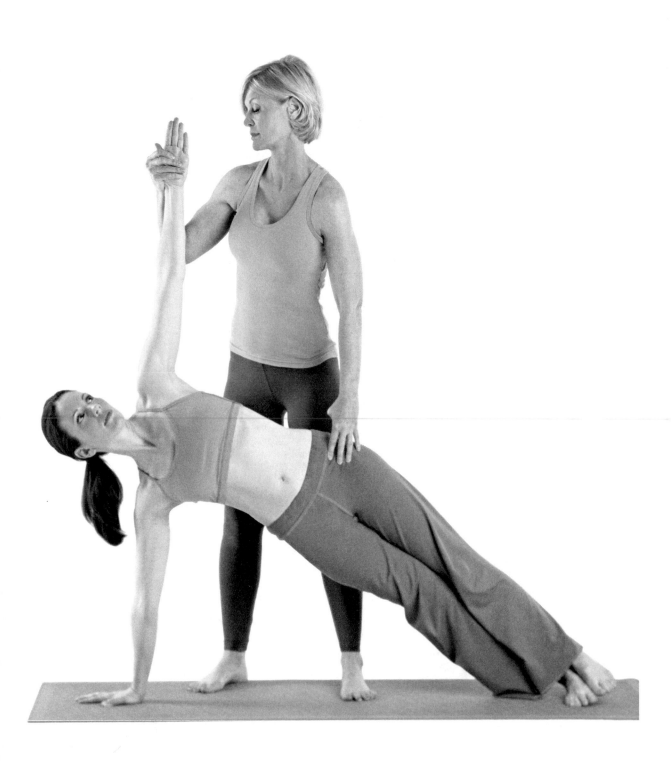

chapter 6

Arms

Are You Armed?

One of the first changes you will notice when you start doing yoga is your arms. Lately, it seems like "yoga arms" are the "in" thing for women. If you are a guy, you have a totally different experience when it comes to your arms and yoga. Most guys already have nice strong-looking arms from lifting weights. So instead, as a guy you might be thinking, "How can these skinny women hold Plank pose effortlessly and I'm dying here?" If your arms are shaking when you are holding simple poses, don't worry. You have to realize that you are holding up all of your body weight. How often do you curl 150 pounds or more? In yoga you are using what are called intrinsic muscles. These are the little internal muscles that you don't see under your skin because they are covered by bigger muscles. That's why body builders have such a hard time with yoga. They often focus on larger muscle groups—you know, the "showy" ones like the biceps.

How Do the Arms Work?

Here's how the arms work. The arm itself is made up of two bones: the long humerus bone and the forearm bones (the radius and the ulna), which are connected by the elbow. These two bones of the arm are attachment points for the medial and lateral collateral ligaments that hold the humerus to the radius and ulna. The muscles of the arm can bend and extend the elbow and rotate the palm up and down. In the forearm, the muscles can also flex; by *extending*, the body part is brought away from the body, and by *adducting*, the body part is brought toward the body. The biceps muscles have two tendons that

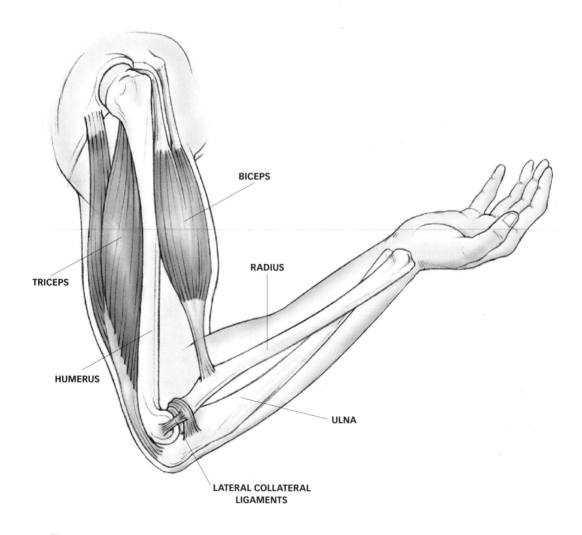

BICEPS

TRICEPS

RADIUS

HUMERUS

ULNA

LATERAL COLLATERAL
LIGAMENTS

attach in different places and also to two different muscles. These two muscles join together to share a common tendon in the forearm. The same is true for the triceps, except that it originates from three tendons and has three different heads that join together for a common tendon in the elbow.

Common Injuries of the Arms

Most of these injuries are "overuse" injuries. As the name implies, you are using that part of your arm too much. Overuse injuries occur when stress is placed on a joint or other tissue, often by "overdoing" an activity or repeating the same activity. Common injuries include:

Tennis elbow: This condition, also called tendinitis, involves inflammation of the tendon that connects the muscles of the forearm, wrist, and hand to the upper arm at the elbow. The tendon on the bony outside part of the elbow (the epicondyle) is most often irritated by overuse during physical activity.

Elbow bursitis: In elbow or olecranon bursitis, repetitive movement causes fluid to collect in the bursa that lies behind the elbow. A bursa is a slippery, sac-like tissue that cushions and lubricates the joint area between one bone and another bone, a tendon, or the skin. It normally allows smooth movement around bone, such as the point behind the elbow. When a bursa becomes inflamed, the sac fills with fluid. This can cause pain and a noticeable swelling behind the elbow. You will find bursa at any area of the body where muscles and tendons glide over bones.

Stress fractures: Stress fractures are hairline cracks in bones. Injuries to the arms can be sudden and may be caused by a direct blow, such as from boxing; by sustaining a fall; or by twisting, jerking, jamming, or bending your arm beyond its range of motion. In this case the pain is sudden and sometimes severe. Bruising and swelling may develop soon after the injury.

Bruises: Bruises (also known as contusions) occur when small blood vessels under the skin tear or rupture, often from a twist, bump, or fall. Blood leaks into tissues under the skin and causes a black-and-blue color.

Strains: Strains, or pulled muscles, may be minor (such as an overstretched muscle) or severe (such as a torn muscle or tendon). Strains are caused by overstretching muscles.

Symptoms may include, depending on how severe:

■ Pain and tenderness that is worse with movement

■ Swelling and bruising

■ Normal or limited muscle movement

■ A bulge or deformity at the site of a complete tear

Fractures: Broken bones may occur when a bone is twisted, struck directly, or used to brace against a fall.

Dislocations: A dislocation occurs when a bone is pulled or pushed out of place. This can happen in joints such as the elbow. A dislocation may be caused by a direct blow to the joint, a fall, or a sudden twisting movement. Everyday activities may cause this injury if a person has unstable joints.

POSES TO HELP YOUR ARMS:

1. Plank pose

2. Four-Limbed Staff pose

3. Side Arm Balance pose

4. Crow pose

Plank Pose

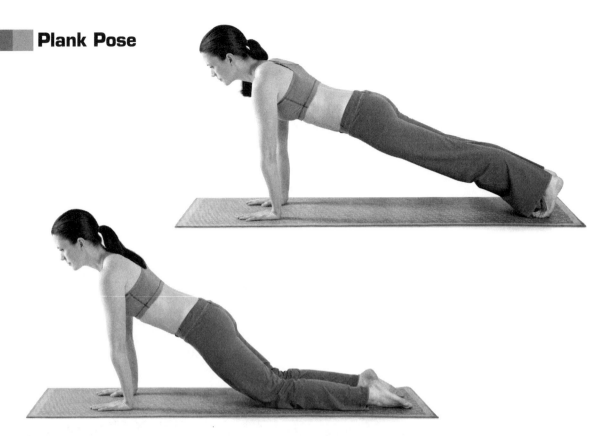

Benefits Plank is a great pose for both your arms and your core strength. When you are doing this pose you are getting a dual workout.

How do you get into this pose?

- Come down to the floor on your hands and knees.
- Bring your hands to about shoulder-distance apart.
- Spread your fingers wide.
- Step back to the point at which you are in what looks like the top of a push-up.
- Make sure your wrists are in line with your shoulders.
- Be as "flat as a board."

- Look straight down between your hands.
- Hold for 30 seconds to 1 minute.

Modify the Pose To make this pose easier, drop down to your knees. Do this until you build enough upper-body strength to hold this pose. To make this pose harder, lift your right leg and hold it up for 30 seconds, then switch legs.

Level of Difficulty Plank looks easy, but it is definitely a hard pose to hold. I would give it an 8.

QUICK-FIX TIP **Don't let your lower back sink in Plank. I see that a lot in new students. If you can't hold the pose correctly, then just modify it as noted above.**

Four-Limbed Staff Pose

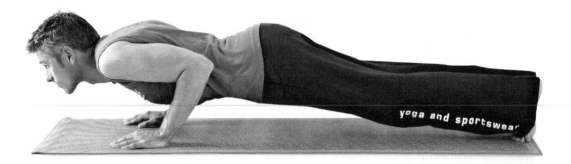

Benefits This pose really takes some upper body and core strength. It strengthens your arms.

How do you get into this pose?

- Come to Plank pose (see preceding page).
- Slowly lower down toward the floor and try to hover 6 inches from the floor.

- Don't let your shoulders drop lower than your elbows.
- Keep your elbows into your sides.
- Hold for 30 seconds to 1 minute. When you can hold it for 1 minute, you are a "pro."
- Either push yourself back up to Plank or lower yourself to the floor.

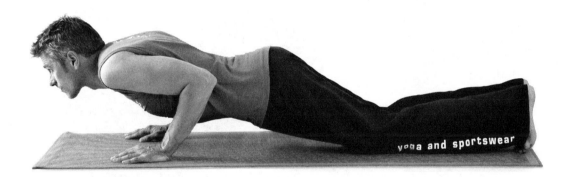

Modify the Pose Drop your knees to the ground.

Level of Difficulty This is a hard pose! I'll give it a 9.

QUICK-FIX TIP Keep the elbows tucked into your body; this protects your shoulders in this pose.

Side Arm Balance Pose

Benefits This pose strengthens the arms and spine. By using your own body weight as resistance in this pose, you can tone not only your arms but your core as well. Working on balance, which engages your core strength, allows you to use all your muscles in this pose.

How do you get into this pose?

- From Plank, bring your right hand underneath your face.
- Shift your weight onto your right hand and lift your left arm up to the ceiling.
- Stack your feet, legs, and hips on top of each other.
- Keep your feet flexed.

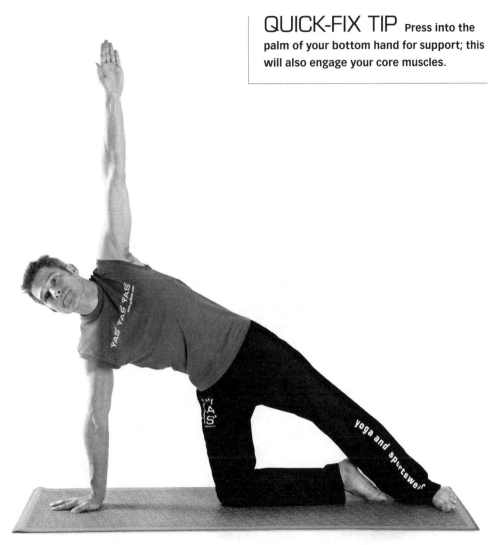

QUICK-FIX TIP Press into the palm of your bottom hand for support; this will also engage your core muscles.

- Lift your hips high by firmly pressing your bottom palm into the ground.

- Hold for 30 seconds and then come back to Plank.

- Switch sides.

- Shift your weight onto your left hand and then bring your right arm to the ceiling.

- Stack your feet on top of each other.

- Hold for 30 seconds.

- Come back to Plank.

- Switch sides.

Modify the Pose If this is a challenging pose for you, drop your bottom knee to the floor.

Level of Difficulty This pose is challenging because it takes not only arm strength but a good amount of core strength—I would rate this at least an 8.

Crow Pose

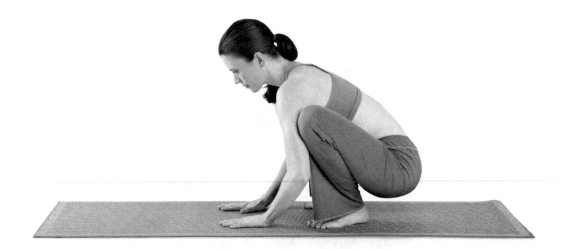

Benefits Crow pose is not an easy pose. It takes not only arm strength but core strength as well. It strengthens the wrists, forearms, and core while improving your overall balance. This is one of those poses that you either love or hate. My students always complain about having to do this pose in class, but I know they secretly practice it at home. When you do finally get this pose, you'll feel a major sense of accomplishment!

How do you get into this pose?

- Squat down.
- Bring your hands between your feet.
- Spread your fingers wide. (Your hands are the feet of your Crow.)
- Bend your elbows.
- Place your knees on your bent forearms.
- Lean forward, balancing your body weight on your triceps.

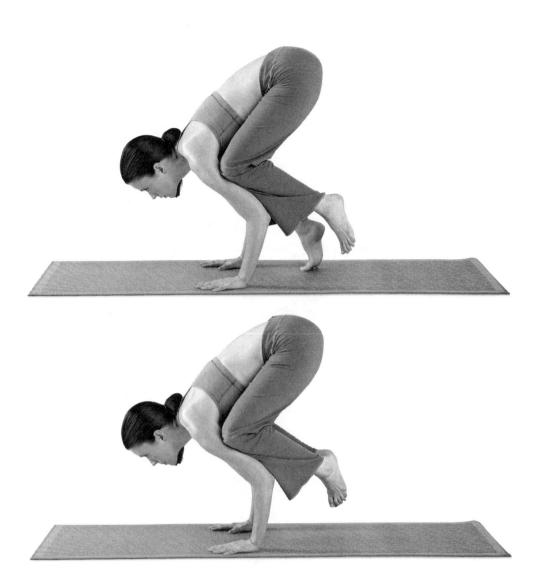

- Lift your toes off the floor.
- Try to keep your head up.

Modify the Pose At first this pose may seem a little scary, so just keep the toes of one foot on the floor to help you with your balance.

Level of Difficulty Crow pose might be a 10 until you master the right "balance" of arm and core strength it takes to do it. I would rate it a 9.

QUICK-FIX TIP Keep your head up; otherwise you will fall forward on your face. Don't worry if you fall—you don't have too far to go. Just remember to "tuck and roll."

"Yoga for Your Arms" Workout Routine: 8 Minutes

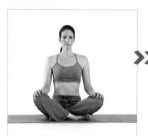 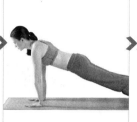 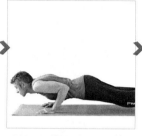 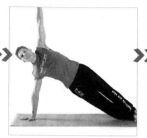

BREATH WORK

Come down to your mat. Sit in an easy cross-legged pose. Sit up tall and close your eyes. Take a minute to center your body and get focused on your arms. Take a deep breath in through your nose and exhale it through your mouth. Repeat this two more times. Each time, try to hold your breath for a few moments before you exhale.

PLANK POSE

Bring your hands about shoulder-distance apart. Step back into what will look like a push-up. Try to hold this pose for at least 30 seconds and work up to 1 minute. If you are finding this pose too hard, just drop down to your knees but keep your arms where they are.

FOUR-LIMBED STAFF POSE

Stay in Plank pose. Slowly lower down and try to hover 6 inches from the floor. Don't let your shoulders drop lower than your elbows. Keep your elbows in at your sides. Hold for 30 seconds to 1 minute. When you can hold it for 1 minute you are a "pro." Either push yourself back up to Plank or lower yourself to the floor and take a break.

SIDE ARM BALANCE POSE

From Plank pose, bring your right hand underneath your face, and then shift your weight onto your right hand. From here, lift your left arm up to the ceiling, stacking your feet, legs, and hips on top of each other. Keep your feet flexed. Lift your hips by firmly pressing your bottom palm into the ground. Hold for 30 seconds and then come back to Plank. Switch sides. Shift your weight onto your left hand and then bring your right arm to the ceiling. Stack your feet on top of each other. Hold for 30 seconds. Then come back to Plank.

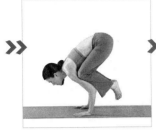 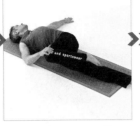 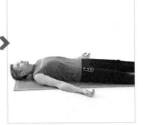

CROW POSE

EASY SPINAL TWIST

CORPSE POSE

Squat down and bring your hands between your feet. With your fingers spread wide, your hands are the feet of your Crow. From here, just bend your elbows and then place your knees on your bent forearms. Try to lean forward, balancing your body weight on your triceps. Lift your toes off the floor. Try to keep your head up. (If you look down, you may tumble over, doing a somersault.) Don't worry if you fall; it happens all the time in class. Remember to "tuck and roll." Hold for 30 seconds to 1 minute. Try this a few times. If you can't get your balance, then just keep the toes of one foot on the floor until you build up enough upper-body strength to hold this pose. It's not an easy pose for anyone, so have patience until you get it.

To release your lower back, bring your left knee into your chest and let your right leg go straight on the floor. Take a deep breath in; on your next exhale, bring the bent knee across your body, keeping your shoulder blades on the floor. Look over your left shoulder to complete this twist. Bring both knees into your chest and then switch sides. Your right knee comes into your chest, and your left leg goes straight. Hold for 45 seconds to 1 minute, then release and bring both knees into your chest. From here we are going into our final pose.

Take a deep breath in; on your exhale, just let your whole body come to the floor. Bring your arms out by your sides with your palms up. Close your eyes and try to let your whole body relax. Notice whether there is any tightness in your body, and relax that area. I want you to take a deep breath in, pretend that you are breathing from your feet, and bring the breath all the way through your body and exhale it all out. Do this two more times, focusing on relaxing your body. Stay here for about 2 minutes to get the maximum benefits. After you are completely relaxed, take a deep breath in through your nose and just "sigh" it out. Bend your knees, roll onto your right side for a few seconds, then push yourself up to a comfortable, easy, cross-legged position like we started with. Bring your hands together in front of your chest, take a deep breath in, and on your exhale bow forward. Take a second to appreciate the fact that you did something good for yourself today. Have an amazing rest of your day!

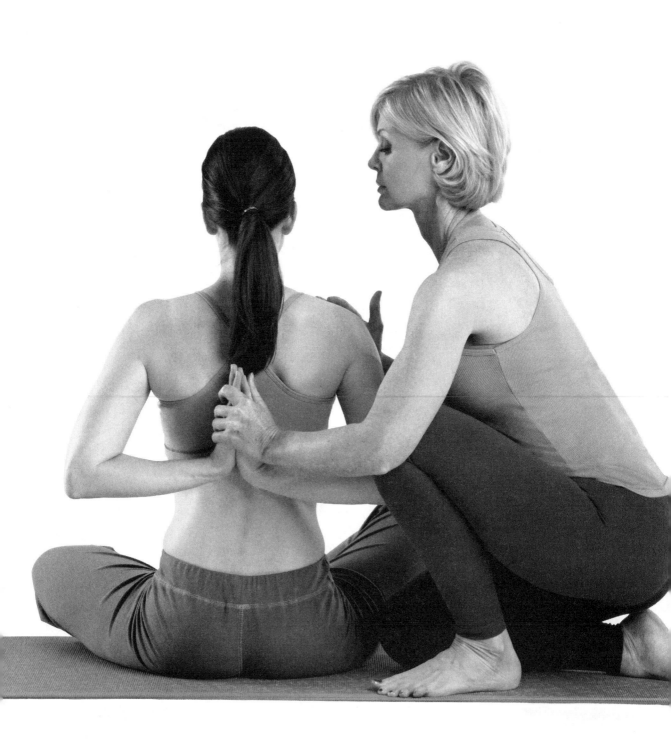

chapter 7

Hands and Wrists

Give Yourself a Pat on the Back

After doing some of the yoga workout routines in this book, you will be able to pat yourself on the back—literally or figuratively, or maybe both! Your hands, like your feet, are a very important part of your body. All of the poses in the "Yoga for Your Arms" workout routine in Chapter 6 work not only your arms but also your hands and wrists. However, I still think it's important to cover the anatomy of the hands and wrists separately from the arms. People who spend the day typing at a computer will find these poses especially rewarding.

How Do the Hands and Wrists Work?

The hands and wrists are a very complicated and fascinating part of the body. The hands consist of many small bones called carpals, metacarpals, and phalanges. The two bones of the lower arm, the radius and the ulna, meet at the hand to form the wrist. Metacarpal bones form the wrist, the carpals form the hand, and the phalanges form the fingers and thumbs. The median and ulnar nerves are the major nerves of the hand, and they run the length of the arm. They transmit electrical impulses to and from the brain to create movement and sensation in your hands.

To understand what causes pain in your hands and wrists, let's take a look at how they function. The wrist helps control the activities of the fingers and thumb by positioning and stabilizing the hand. Most of the wrist's movement occurs at the juncture of the radius, one of the two forearm bones, and several of the carpal bones, deep in the heel of your hand. Some movement also occurs at the junctures between the individual carpal bones. The movements of the wrist include abduction (bending the thumb side of the hand toward the thumb side of the forearm), adduction (bending the little-finger side of the hand toward the little-finger side of the forearm), flexion, and extension.

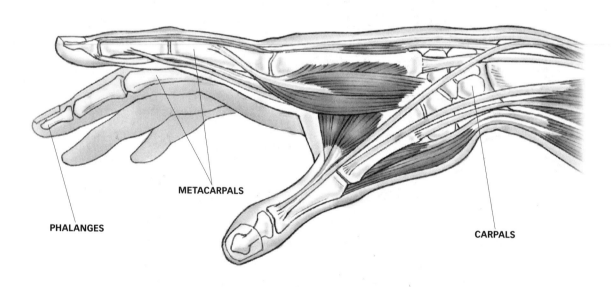

PHALANGES

METACARPALS

CARPALS

In yoga, by far the most important of these—and probably the one most likely to bring you grief—is extension. To feel this wrist movement, sit in a chair with armrests and put one of your forearms on an armrest, palm facing the floor. Bring your hand up, pointing your fingers toward the ceiling. Your wrist is now in extension. If you let your hand hang over the end of the armrest and your fingers point toward the floor, your wrist will be in flexion. Most likely, you spend a lot of time every day with your wrist in mild extension. This position is the one we use most often in daily activities. So your wrist probably spends very little time in full flexion or full extension. Because the wrist, like any other joint, will lose any part of its range of motion that isn't used regularly, most people gradually lose the ability to move easily and safely into full wrist extension (a 90-degree angle between the hand and forearm). The good news is that nothing is better for strengthening your hands and wrists than yoga.

Common Injuries to the Hands/Wrists

Tendonitis: Tendonitis of the wrist is an irritation and swelling of the tissue or "tunnel" that surrounds the tendons of the thumb. Pain in the front of the wrist is a common symptom of tendonitis. Bending and extending the wrist is usually painful; there may be swelling in the wrist. If pain worsens when the hand is made into a fist and the thumb is tucked inside, you probably have tendonitis. Tendonitis of the wrist can be caused by biomechanical problems, injury to the arm, and overuse. The wrist tendons often become inflamed when you start a new activity or exercise. If treated early, pain associated with tendonitis can be alleviated quickly with some anti-inflammatory medication such as ibuprofen.

Carpal tunnel syndrome: This term describes a specific group of symptoms (tingling, numbness, weakness, or pain) in the fingers or hand and occasionally in the lower arm and elbow. These symptoms occur when there is pressure on a nerve (median nerve) within the wrist (carpal tunnel). Carpal tunnel syndrome develops over time as a result of repetitive hand motions that damage muscle and bone in the wrist area. It's an irritation of the synovial membranes around the tendons in the carpal tunnel. This inflammation puts pressure on the median nerve, which travels from the forearm into the hand through a "tunnel" in your wrist. The bottom and sides of this tunnel are formed by wrist bones, while the top of the tunnel is covered by a strong band of connective tissue or ligament. This tunnel also contains nine tendons that connect muscles to bones and allow you to bend your fingers and thumb. These tendons are covered with a lubricating membrane called synovium, which may enlarge and swell under some circumstances. Severe swelling may cause the median nerve to be pressed up against this strong ligament, which may result in numbness, tingling in your hand, clumsiness, or pain, all classic signs of carpal tunnel syndrome. This condition is becoming very common; over 1 million people a year see a doctor for wrist issues.

The good news is that yoga can help reduce the pain of carpal tunnel syndrome. A study published in the *Journal of the American Medical Association* concluded that people who practiced yoga over an 8-week period showed improvement in their condition compared with those who did not do yoga. The poses emphasized in this study focused on opening, stretching, and strengthening the joints of the upper body (see Chapter 6, Arms). However, if you have carpal tunnel syndrome, you should modify the poses that place too much pressure on the wrists. Modifications include doing the pose with closed fists rather than flat palms because this reduces the pressure on the wrists.

SIGNS AND SYMPTOMS OF CARPAL TUNNEL SYNDROME:

- Numbness and tingling in the hands
- Decreased sensation in the thumb and fingers
- Tingling over the wrist
- Pain when holding the wrist in a bent position for a period of time

CAUSES OF CARPAL TUNNEL SYNDROME:

Carpal tunnel syndrome can be caused by anything that irritates the synovial membranes around the tendons of the hands and, in turn, places pressure on the median nerve. Some common causes include:

- Repetitive grasping with the hands/repetitive bending of the wrist and overuse
- Increase in the intensity and duration of exercise (racket sports are common culprits)
- Improper and ill-fitting equipment
- Broken or dislocated bones in the wrist, which produce swelling
- Arthritis, especially the rheumatoid type
- Thyroid gland imbalance
- Diabetes

Wrist sprain: A sprain is a stretched or torn ligament. Ligaments are tissues that connect bones at a joint. Falling, twisting, or getting hit can all cause a sprain. Wrist sprains are common. Symptoms include pain, swelling, bruising, and inability to move your joint. You might feel a pop or tear when the injury happens. Strains can occur suddenly or develop over time. Many people get sprains playing sports.

Broken wrist: When you break your wrist, you probably are talking about a broken scaphoid bone, which is located on the thumb side where the wrist bends. The scaphoid can be identified more easily when the thumb is held in a "hitchhiking" position. A fracture usually results from a fall on an outstretched hand, with the weight landing on the palm. The end of one of the forearm bones—the radius—may also break in this type of fall, depending on the position of the hand when you land. The injury can also occur during sports. Some studies have shown that use of wrist guards during activities such as inline skating and snowboarding can decrease the chance of breaking a bone around the wrist.

Poses That Help Your Hands and Wrists

All the poses that are in Chapter 6, Arms, also work on your hands and wrists. If you are having pain in this area, then this "Yoga for Your Hands and Wrists" workout will be good for you. It's very simple and can be done anywhere. You can do it at your computer at work or at home. Because so many people have issues with their wrists, you may want to do this routine even if your wrists are fine. Strengthening your wrists will help to safeguard against injury. What do you do in a yoga class to modify the typical yoga poses if you have hand or wrist issues? In poses such as Plank, which you did in Chapter 6, you would drop down to your knees to take about 80% of the pressure off your wrists. In a pose such as Downward-Facing Dog, you can shift your weight back into the heels. I always tell my students that they should be able to lift their hands off the mat in Downward-Facing Dog because this actually requires more core strength. As always, if you have a hand or wrist injury, ask your doctor before you do this or any other exercise.

POSES TO HELP YOUR HANDS AND WRISTS:

1. Wrist Rolls (closed fist)

2. Mountain pose (arms above and clasped)

3. Reverse Prayer pose

4. Plank pose (up against a wall)

5. Four-Limbed Staff pose (up against a wall)

Wrist Rolls (Closed Fist)

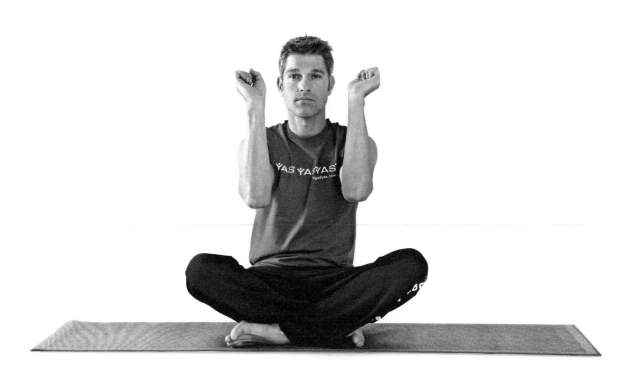

Benefits This pose stretches your wrists and brings circulation into your hands.

How do you get into this pose?

■ Do this pose while sitting at your desk.

■ Close your hands into a fist.

■ Roll your hands from your wrist, to the left and then to the right.

■ Do this for 30 to 45 seconds each way.

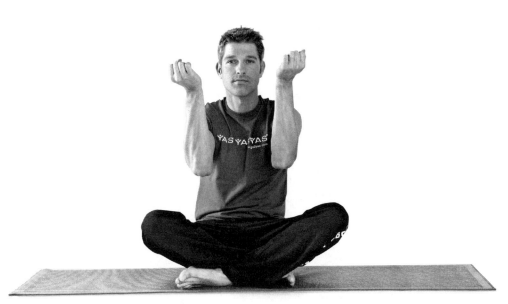

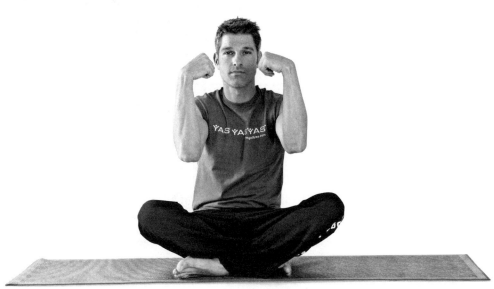

Modify the Pose Do this pose with your fingers open.

Level of Difficulty Very easy—I would give it a 2. Just remember to take it easy if you have a wrist injury.

QUICK-FIX TIP You just want to get some circulation into your hands and wrists, so don't force this.

Mountain Pose (Arms Above and Clasped)

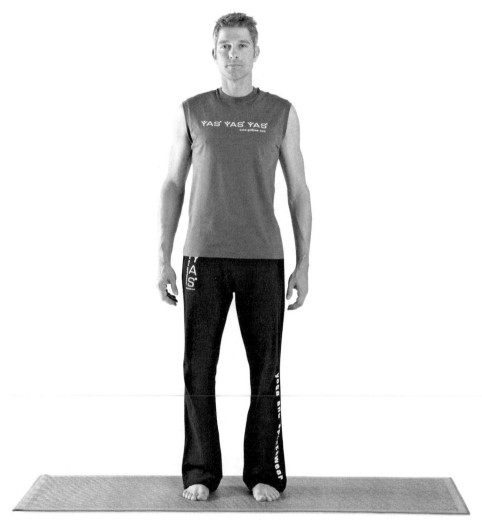

Benefits This pose stretches out your fingers. It's a good pose to do if you have been at your computer for a long time.

How do you get into this pose?

■ Stand up straight with your hips tucked underneath you.

■ Bring your hands over your head.

■ Clasp your hands together.

■ Bring your palms to the ceiling.

■ Hold for 45 seconds to 1 minute.

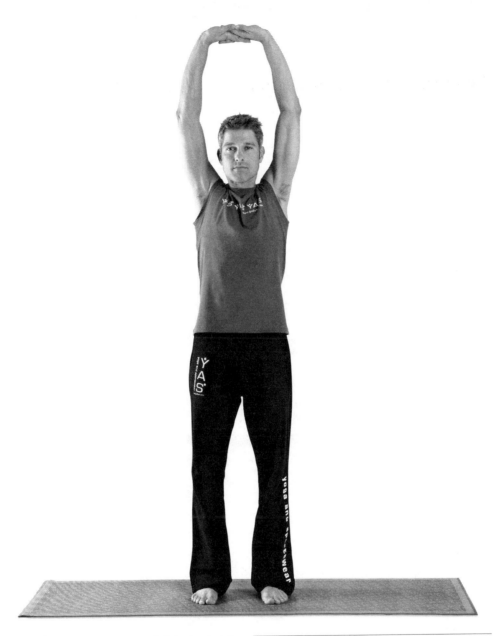

Modify the Pose To get a full-body stretch, do this pose standing instead of seated at your desk.

Level of Difficulty Fairly easy. I would give it a 4.5, but just think of it as a mini-break from work.

QUICK-FIX TIP **Try to do this pose every day whether you think you need to or not. It will not only stretch out your fingers after a lot of typing but also stretch out your neck muscles.**

Reverse Prayer Pose

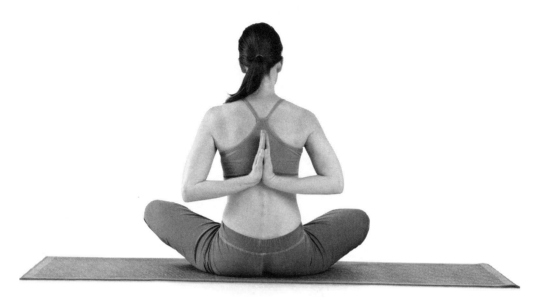

Benefits This pose will not only stretch out your wrists but also strengthen your fingers.

How do you get into this pose?

- Do this pose either seated or standing.
- Bring your hands behind your back.
- Press your hands together.
- Hold for 30 to 45 seconds, then release.
- Repeat three times.

Modify the Pose Instead of doing this pose behind your back, just bring your hands together in front of your chest and press your hands together firmly.

Level of Difficulty This one is a little more difficult. It will take some flexibility in your shoulders to get your hands behind your back, so I would give it a 6.

QUICK-FIX TIP Press into the pinky side of your hands, and as your wrists and hands stretch, see if you can bring your hands up your back, closer to your shoulders.

Plank Pose (Up Against a Wall)

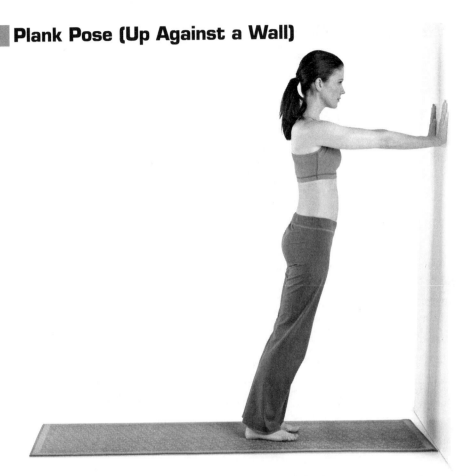

Benefits This pose strengthens and stretches the muscles in the hands and wrists.

How do you get into this pose?

- Stand facing a wall, about arms-length away.
- Place your hands on the wall with your fingers spread wide.
- Lean into your hands.
- Hold for 45 seconds to 1 minute.

Modify the Pose To make this pose harder, walk your feet away from the wall. That way you are using more of your body weight to press into the wall with your hands.

Level of Difficulty This is an easy pose; I would rate it a 4.5.

QUICK-FIX TIP Make sure your fingers are spread wide and that all of them are pressing into the wall.

Four-Limbed Staff Pose (Up Against a Wall)

Benefits This pose works on not only the strength in your hands but also the flexion of your wrists.

How do you get into this pose?

- From Plank pose against a wall (see preceding pose), bend your elbows.
- Keep your elbows into your body.
- Allow your body to come as close to the wall as it can.
- Hold for 30 to 45 seconds.
- Repeat three times.

Modify the Pose To make this pose easier, don't lower yourself as close to the wall. To make it harder, walk your feet a little farther from the wall.

Level of Difficulty In general this is an easy pose, so I would rate it a 5.

QUICK-FIX TIP I suggest you do this pose a few times a day if you work in an office. Use it as a mini-break for your hands and wrists. Focus on releasing your shoulders as well.

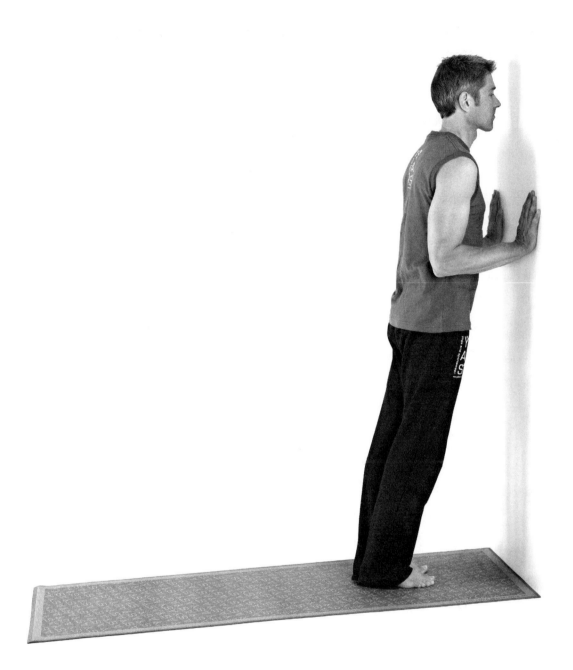

"Yoga for Your Hands and Wrists" Workout Routine: 8 Minutes

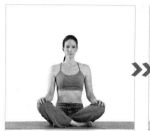 >> 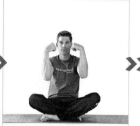 >> 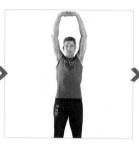 >> 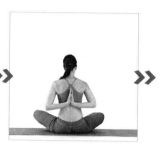 >>

BREATH WORK

WRIST ROLLS (CLOSED FIST)

MOUNTAIN POSE (ARMS ABOVE AND CLASPED)

REVERSE PRAYER POSE

Since you are probably doing this at your desk, instead of coming to the floor, just sit up tall at your desk and close your eyes. We are going to take a minute to center your body and get you focused on your hands and wrists. Take a deep breath in through your nose and exhale it through your mouth. Repeat this two more times. Each time try to hold your breath for a few moments before you exhale.

Stay seated and bring your arms out in front of you with your hands in a fist. Take a deep breath in; on your exhale, start to roll your fists to the right for 30 to 45 seconds and then repeat going to the left.

You can do this pose seated or, if you feel like it, standing up. Take a deep breath in, and on your exhale bring your arms over your head. Clasp your hands together and then bring your palms to the ceiling. Hold this pose for 45 seconds to 1 minute. You can lean to your right and then to your left to get an extra stretch.

If you decide to stand for Mountain pose, stay standing. Take a deep breath in, and on your exhale bring your hands behind your back in a prayer position. Try to press into the pinky side on your hand. Hold for 30 to 45 seconds. If this is too hard, bring your hands in front of your chest in a prayer position and just press your hands together.

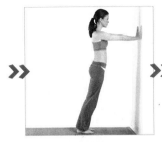

**PLANK POSE
(UP AGAINST A WALL)**

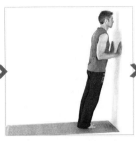

**FOUR-LIMBED STAFF POSE
(UP AGAINST A WALL)**

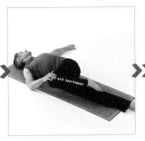

EASY SPINAL TWIST

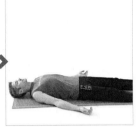

CORPSE POSE

If you have been sitting, take a break from your chair and go up to a wall. You want to be about arms-length from the wall. Place both hands up against the wall with your fingers spread wide. From here, just lean into the wall to build strength in your hands. Hold for 45 seconds to 1 minute. To make this more challenging, walk your feet a little farther away from the wall.

Stay in Plank pose up against a wall. Take a deep breath in; on your exhale, bend your elbows and bring your nose to the wall. Hold for 30 to 45 seconds and then push away, coming back to Plank. Do this three times.

Come down to the floor and lie on your back. If you are doing this at work, make sure you lie down on a rug or bring your yoga mat to work. Finish this sequence with the Easy Spinal Twist to release your lower back before you hop back on your computer. Bring both knees into your chest. Then straighten your right leg and keep your left knee at your chest. Take a deep breath in; on your exhale, bring the bent knee across your body, keeping your shoulder blades on the floor. Look over your left shoulder to complete your twist. Bring both knees into your chest and then switch sides; the right knee comes into your chest, and the left leg goes straight. Bring your knee across your body and hold for 45 seconds to 1 minute. Release and bring both knees into your chest.

From here we are going into our final pose, Corpse. Take a deep breath in; on your exhale, just let your whole body come down to the floor. Bring your arms out by your sides with your palms up; we are going to end this workout like we started it, with a little breath work. Close your eyes, and try to let your whole body relax. Notice whether there is any tightness in your body, and relax that area. I want you to take a deep breath in, pretend that you are breathing from your feet, and bring the breath all the way through your body and exhale all the breath out. Do this two more times, focusing on relaxing your body. Stay here for about 2 minutes to get the maximum benefits. After you are completely relaxed, take a deep breath in through your nose and just "sigh" it out. Bend your knees, roll onto your right side for a few seconds, then push yourself up to a comfortable, easy, cross-legged position. Bring your hands together in front of your chest, take a deep breath in, and on your exhale bow forward. Take a second to appreciate the fact that you did something good for yourself today!

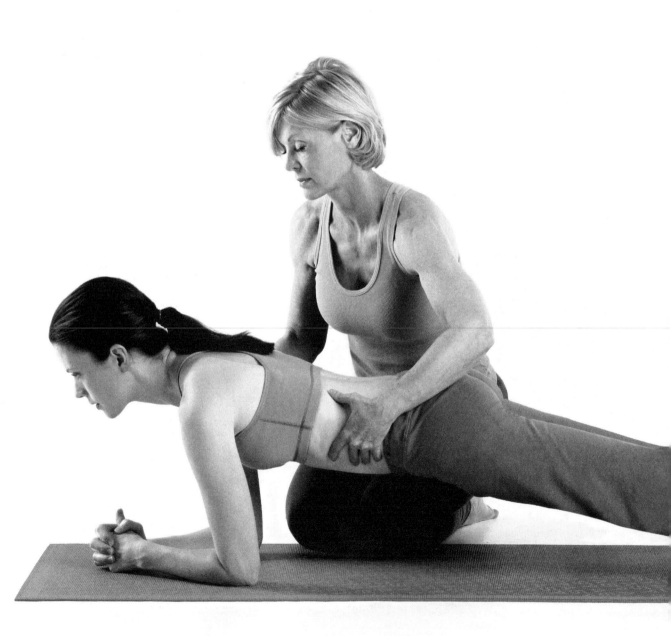

chapter 8

Core/Abs

It's NOT All about Having a Six-Pack

Yoga is all about "core strength" because most of the poses in yoga work all the intrinsic muscles that make up your core. When you think about your core/abs, most of the time you are thinking "six-pack." But the core is a lot more than a six-pack; it consists of your whole torso. Core strength is one of the main benefits of doing yoga. The core is your "center of power." Everything starts with your core, especially in sports—that's why we need to keep it strong. When your core is strong, you feel more confident. There are a lot of reasons you want to keep your core strong. One of the main reasons, besides looking good in your bathing suit, is that a strong core protects your lower back from injuries. Whether you are playing competitive sports or just getting out of bed in the morning, everything starts with your core.

How Do the Core/Abs Work?

Core strength is the development of the abdominal and back muscles that surround your torso. The core muscles stabilize the body and represent a link between your legs and arms. These muscles include all the muscles in your torso, not only those in your abdominals and back but also the ones in your pelvic floor and hips. Many of your core muscles can't be seen because they're buried underneath other larger muscles. These buried muscles are the intrinsic muscles. So it's not just about the six-pack, the big muscle group on the top; it's also about the transverse abdominis, which is underneath your rectus abdominis (that is, the six-pack) and hugs the whole area below your belly button. The rectus abdominis is sitting on top. The transverse abdominis is underneath, keeping your posture upright and protecting your internal organs. You can't see the erector spinae, either; it's behind you, supporting your back. All of these muscles work together to keep your torso stable while your arms and legs

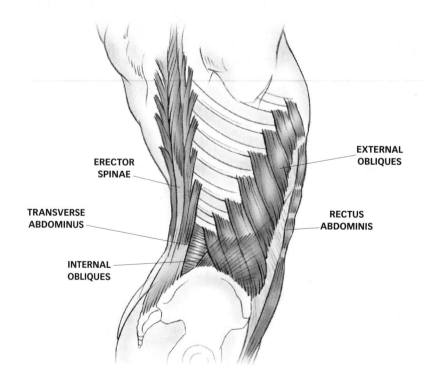

ERECTOR
SPINAE

EXTERNAL
OBLIQUES

TRANSVERSE
ABDOMINUS

RECTUS
ABDOMINIS

INTERNAL
OBLIQUES

are moving. So you can see why strong core muscles keep your back healthy. They also hold your body upright and improve your balance. If the core muscles are weak, your body doesn't work as effectively, and other muscles have to compensate for them. This can result in injuries such as a twisted knee, a pulled shoulder, or a bad back. If you play sports, a strong core will help you with your "power moves," and your whole body will function more effectively. A strong core even helps you breathe better, which improves your oxygen supply in sports, and some of the intercostals (the muscles between the ribs) help with exhalation. If the muscles are short, usually because of poor breathing patterns or prolonged slumping, they limit the chest opening. Muscles become short for two reasons. Either they are regularly worked hard (like the abs of someone who does a lot of sit-ups) and are not stretched, or they are regularly placed in a shortened position (like those of someone sitting for long periods of time) and are not stretched. In either case, yoga is the key to improvement.

Common Injuries of the Core/Abs

Lower back injuries: This is not exactly an injury of your core, but it can occur because your core is weak (the leading cause of back problems). If you are having lower back issues, see Chapter 9, Lower Back.

Abdominal muscle strain: Also called a pulled abdominal muscle, it's an injury to one of the muscles of the abdominals. Normally a muscle strain occurs when the muscle is stretched too far. When this occurs, the muscle fibers are torn. Most commonly, a strain causes microscopic tears within the muscle, but occasionally, in severe injuries, the muscle can rupture from its attachment.

Hernia: A hernia is an opening or weakness in the abdominals. This causes a bulging of the abdominal wall, which is usually noticeable when the abdominal muscles are tightened. This increases the pressure in the abdomen. Even the thought of this should be enough to get you to do the following poses.

> **POSES TO HELP YOUR CORE/ABS:**
> **1.** Plank pose
> **2.** Reverse Hover (aka Four-Legged Staff) pose or Low Push-Up
> **3.** Dolphin pose (with movement)
> **4.** Boat pose
> **5.** Yoga Bicycle pose
> **6.** Windshield Wiper pose

Plank Pose

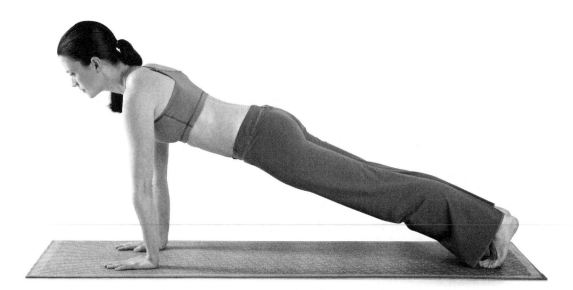

Benefits This pose strengthens your arms, wrists, and back while strengthening the core. I do a lot of Planks in my classes. It's one of my favorite poses because you get a lot of "bang for your buck."

How do you get into this pose?

■ Come down to the floor on all fours and step back so you are in an upper push-up position.

■ Bring your hands directly under your

shoulders, stacking your shoulders, elbows, and wrists in one line.

■ Tuck your toes under and come up on the balls of your feet. Make sure your feet are hip-distance apart.

■ Spread your fingers wide and look down between your hands.

■ Engage your legs; lift the front of your thighs and press back through your heels.

■ Use your core strength here to support yourself.

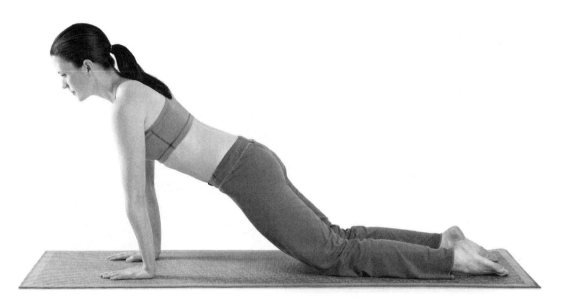

- This pose works your arms, but right now what is keeping you in this pose is your core strength.
- Hold for 30 seconds to 1 minute.

Modify the Pose If you cannot hold yourself up in the pose, then drop down to your knees, but keep your arms right where they were.

Level of Difficulty This is an 8. Don't worry, you'll develop core strength over time and this pose will become easier.

QUICK-FIX TIP A common mistake I see students make in this pose is having their hands too far apart. Make sure your shoulders, elbows, and wrists are in one line.

Reverse Hover (Four-Legged Staff) Pose or Low Push-Up

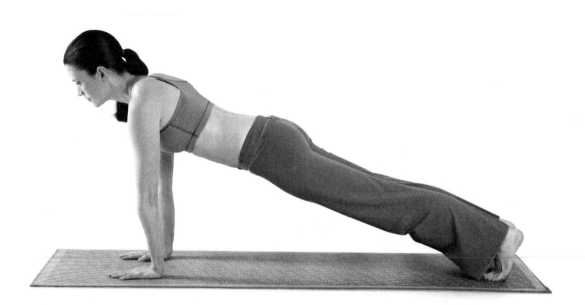

Benefits This pose works on your biceps, triceps, shoulders, and chest muscles, as well as your core/abs.

QUICK-FIX TIP **Keep your elbows in, by your sides, to protect your shoulders.**

How do you get into this pose?

■ Start in Plank.

■ Lower down by bending your elbows so that your body rests about 5 inches off the ground.

■ Try to keep your shoulders in line with your elbows.

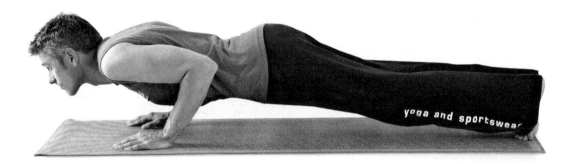

- Your elbows should be at a 90-degree angle.
- Hold this position for 30 seconds. Work up to 1 minute if you want to really challenge yourself!

Modify the Pose If this pose is too challenging, drop your knees to the ground but keep your arms where they are. If you're worn out from your run or workout, you can use this modification until you build up enough upper-body strength.

Level of Difficulty Now this pose is definitely a 9.5. It's really hard to hold!

Dolphin Pose

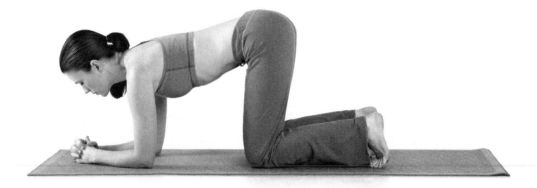

Benefits This is another one of those poses that yoga magazines, books, and Web sites say does everything from preventing osteoporosis to curing depression, insomnia, high blood pressure, and flat feet. Let's take a look at Dolphin pose and see why that might be the case, or at least the physical benefits of this pose that would affect these symptoms. Preventing osteoporosis? Hmm, it strengthens your core, which protects your lower back. That might be "stretching" it, no pun intended. Depression? It's not an easy pose to do; if you have the energy to do this pose, then you're probably not depressed. Insomnia? Well, doing yoga in general helps with sleep. Flat feet? You are up on your toes with this pose; again, though, that seems to be stretching things!

QUICK-FIX TIP **The slower you go, the more challenging this pose and the more muscles you use. So if you want to challenge yourself, slow it down.**

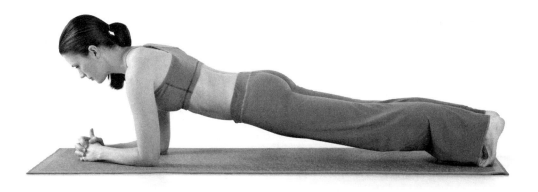

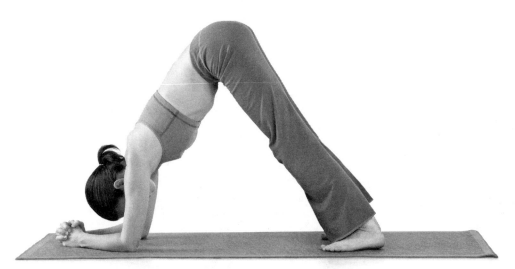

How do you get into this pose?

- Come down to the floor on your knees.
- Drop your forearms to the ground and interlace your fingers.
- Press your forearms firmly into the ground, lengthening your spine.
- Elbows should be as wide apart as your shoulders.
- If you can, straighten your legs, raising your hips high with your chest open.
- Look up and move your chest forward so your face hovers right over your hands.
- Hold here for a few seconds and then press back.
- Try not to collapse into your shoulders, lowering your chin just past your hands.
- Repeat five to 10 times, slowly!

Modify the Pose Instead of shifting your weight out over your hands, just hold Dolphin—no movement.

Level of Difficulty This is a very challenging pose. I would give it an 8.5.

Boat Pose

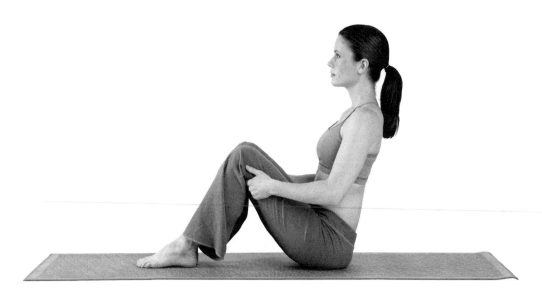

Benefits This pose is great for your core muscles. It strengthens your abs, hip flexors, and lower back.

How do you get into this pose?

- Come down to the floor with your legs out in front of you.
- Bring your arms behind you and press your palms into the floor for support.
- Lean slightly back.

- Bend your knees and bring your legs off the floor.
- Balance on your tailbone.
- Try to straighten your legs; if you can't, it's no big deal—just keep your knees bent for now.
- Bring your arms alongside the outside of your legs.
- Hold for 30 seconds to 1 minute.

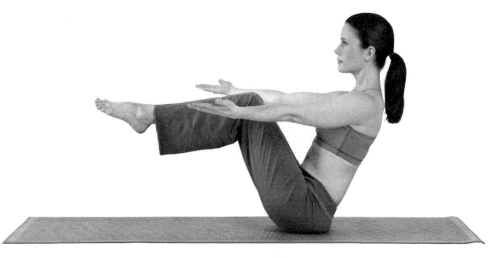

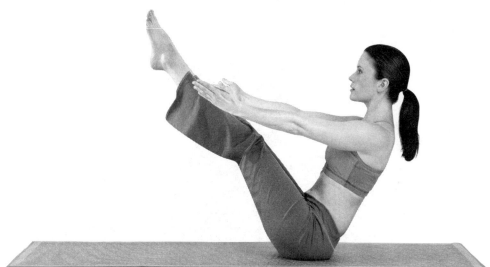

Modify the Pose To make this pose a little easier, keep your hands on the floor behind you for support.

Level of Difficulty Yikes, this is a hard one. I would rate it at least a 9.

QUICK-FIX TIP You can use a strap or a towel to help you with this pose. Loop the strap around the soles of your feet. Make sure you keep your back flat.

Yoga Bicycle Pose

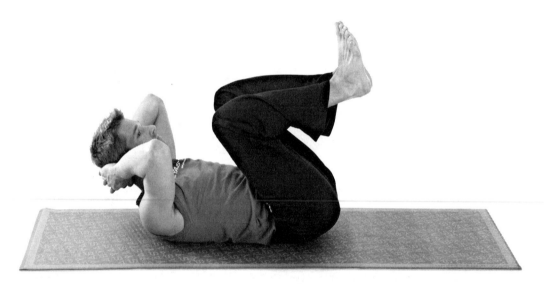

Benefits This pose works the lower abs.

QUICK-FIX TIP The slower you go, the more challenging this pose is and the more muscles you use. Make sure you are breathing. Exhale as you twist (you want to do this in every pose).

How do you get into the pose?

- Lie down on your back.
- Bring your knees to your chest.
- Keeping your knees bent, bring your left elbow to your right knee.
- Let your left leg go straight.
- Switch sides, just like riding a bike.
- Do 10 of these, alternating sides. Keep it slow.

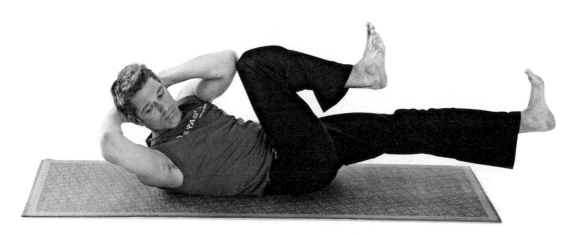

Modify the Pose To make this even more challenging, pause for a few seconds when your elbow touches your knee, then switch sides.

Level of Difficulty This is a pretty easy pose—I would give it a 5.

Windshield Wiper Pose

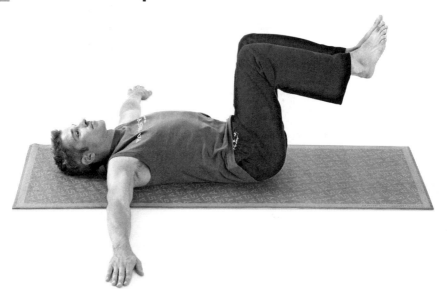

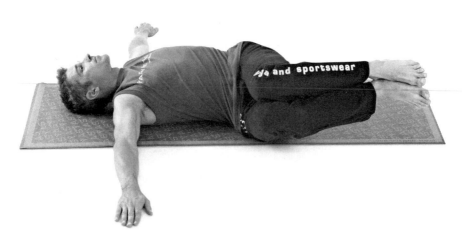

Benefits This pose is great for your obliques, which are located on the sides of your torso.

How do you get into the pose?

- Lie on the floor on your back.
- Bring your knees to a 45-degree angle. Keep your knees bent.
- Bring your arms straight out at your shoulders, palms down on the ground for support.
- Slowly lower your legs to the right side.
- Hover a couple of inches from the ground.

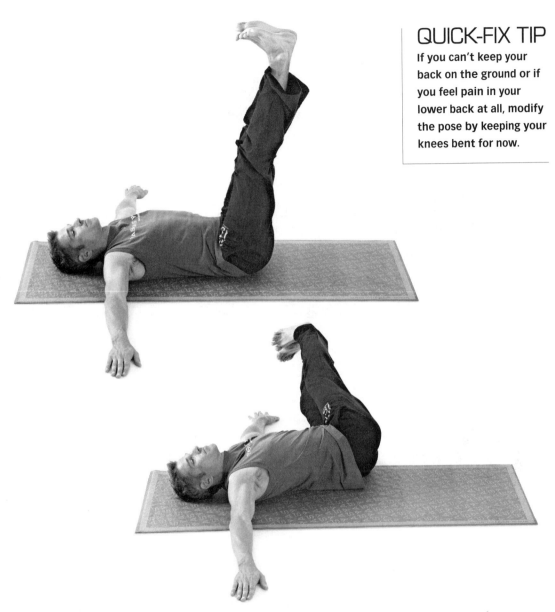

QUICK-FIX TIP

If you can't keep your back on the ground or if you feel pain in your lower back at all, modify the pose by keeping your knees bent for now.

- Bring your legs back up to center, then switch sides.
- Keep your legs together.
- Keep your back on the floor.
- Do 10 of these, five on each side.

Modify the Pose If this is easy for you, straighten your legs. Try to keep as much of your back on the ground as you can. This pose is for the sides of your body, your obliques.

Level of Difficulty This pose is pretty easy, so I would rate it a 5.

"Yoga for Your Core/Abs" Workout Routine: 10 Minutes

Now this is not an easy workout—these poses will definitely challenge you! Don't worry if you can't do them all perfectly, or if you can't do some of them at all at this point. With time you will build up the core strength to do the whole routine. I will give you some modifications to the more challenging poses.

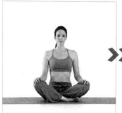 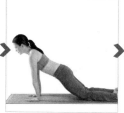 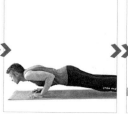 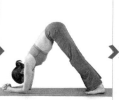 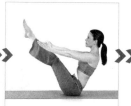

BREATH WORK	PLANK POSE	HOVER POSE	DOLPHIN POSE	BOAT POSE

Come down to your mat if you have one. Sit in an easy cross-legged pose. Sit up tall and close your eyes. Take a minute to center your body and get yourself focused on your core/abs. Take a deep breath in through your nose and exhale it through your mouth. We're going to do this two more times. Each time, try to hold your breath for a few moments before you exhale.

From here I want you to come to all fours. Bring your hands about shoulder-distance apart with your fingers spread wide. Step your feet back and come to the top of a push-up. This is a challenging pose all on its own; I want you to try to hold this pose for 45 seconds to 1 minute. Right now you are working 20% arms and 80% core.

From here, lower all the way to the floor. Once you are down, push yourself up and hover 6 inches from the floor. I want you to try this two more times.

Drop your knees to the mat; bring your elbows and forearms on the floor about shoulder-distance apart. Clasp your hands together, tuck your toes back, and push yourself back to Downward-Facing Dog position, but with your elbows on the floor. Make sure you are on a padded surface. Now this may be as far as you go; that's okay, just stay here and hold this pose for 30 to 45 seconds. If you want to challenge yourself, take a deep breath in and on your next exhale shift your weight forward, bringing your chin right above your hands. Then shift your weight back. Do this five times. Remember to breathe. Drop down to your knees to take a mini-break. Shift your weight on to your side and then come to a seated position for Boat pose.

Personally I find this pose to be difficult. I broke my tailbone in a riding accident, so for me balancing on my tailbone is not easy. Bring your legs together with your knees bent and your feet on the ground. Bring your feet up to the point where they are at knee level. Bring your arms out alongside your knees, with your palms facing each other. Now this may be as far as you go, but if this pose is easy for you then straighten your legs to a wide "V" shape. Hold for about 30 seconds to 1 minute. Then hug your knees into your chest and roll down onto your back. Rock side to side to release your lower back and take a mini-break.

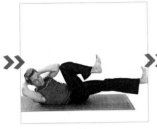 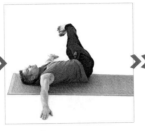 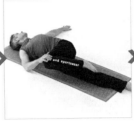 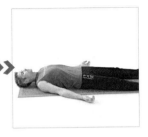

YOGA BICYCLE POSE

Keep your knees bent, bring your hands underneath your head, take a deep breath in, and on your exhale bring your left elbow to your right knee. Hold it for 10 seconds, then switch sides. Take a deep breath in; on your exhale, bring your right elbow to your left knee. I want you to do 10 of these, five on each side. The slower you go in this pose the harder it is, so if you really want to challenge yourself, slow it down. When you are done with that, hug your knees into your chest and rock side to side to release your lower back.

WINDSHIELD WIPER POSE

I want you to keep your knees bent for now. Bring your arms straight out at shoulder level, with your palms facing the floor. You want your palms down so you have some leverage in this pose; this helps you keep your lower back on the ground. Bring your knees to the right side of your body and hover a few inches off the floor. Then switch sides. If this happens to be an easy pose for you, go ahead and straighten your legs. If you do decide to try this, make sure your back is on the ground. You shouldn't feel this in your lower back; this pose is working on what is called your obliques (basically the sides of your torso). I want you to do this 10 times, five on each side. Remember: slow, slow, slow! From here, just hug your knees into your chest and rock side to side to release your lower back.

EASY SPINAL TWIST

To release your lower back, bring your left knee into your chest and let your right leg go straight on the floor. Take a deep breath in; on your exhale, bring the bent knee across your body, keeping your shoulder blades on the floor. Look over your left shoulder to complete your twist. Bring both knees into your chest and then switch sides; the right knee comes into your chest, and the left leg goes straight. Hold for 45 seconds to 1 minute, then release and bring both knees into your chest.

CORPSE POSE

From here we are going into our final pose, Corpse pose. Bring your arms out by your sides with your palms up. Remember, don't skip this part—it helps the body adjust to what you just did and allows the benefits of your routine to sink into your body before you run off. Close your eyes, and try to let your whole body relax. I want you to take a deep breath in, pretend that you are breathing from your feet, and bring the breath all the way through your body and exhale all the breath out. Do this two more times, focusing on relaxing your body. Stay here for about 2 minutes to get the maximum benefits. Bend your knees, roll onto your right side for a few seconds, then push yourself up to a comfortable, easy, cross-legged position like we started with. Take a second to appreciate the fact that you did something good for yourself today. Go out and conquer the world with your newfound core strength!

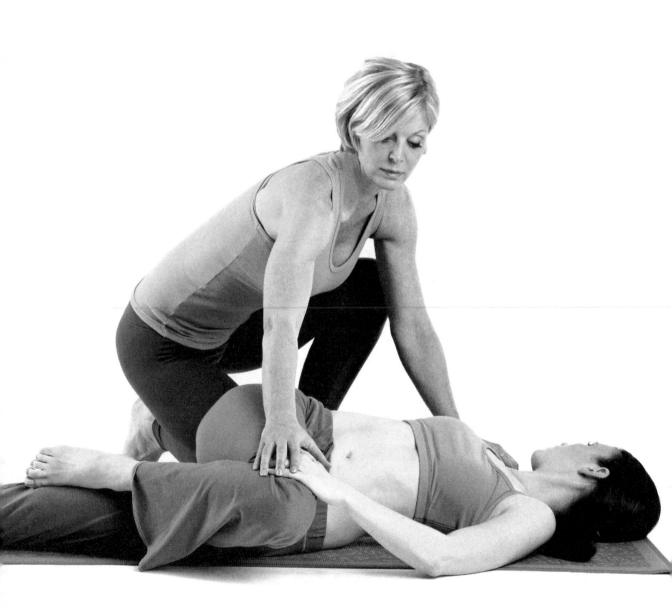

chapter 9

Lower Back

Don't Look Back!

When the muscles in your back become weak, that's normally when your back goes out. The vertebrae in your back are held in place by a lot of small muscles and ligaments, which need to be exercised to keep them in shape. Lower back issues are one of the most common complaints I hear from new students. Usually after they start doing yoga their lower back pain goes away.

There are many reasons for lower back pain. Sometimes it's caused by stress or sitting too long at your desk or in your car. For women, lower back pain can be caused by wearing high heels, or it can occur in new moms picking up their babies. Some women carry their babies on their hip, primarily on one side, which throws their back out. Unfortunately, I see this a lot. In sports, the lower back is affected—say by pounding the pavements while running. With golfing, the stress of the golf swing or walking the course carrying your bag can affect the back (not all of us have the luxury of a caddie!). Other sports-related causes of lower back injury include being hit, usually in contact sports such as football, or stopping and starting quickly, as in tennis or basketball.

If you know your lower back pain is coming from stress, you might want to read Chapter 1, Head. If you know your lower back is bothering you because your core/abs are weak, check out Chapter 8. Of course, if you have severe back pain, make sure to check with your doctor before you try yoga or any other exercise. Some back issues can come from what is called "biomechanical imbalances" in your spine. Doing yoga will be great for your back in this case because it works on not only flexibility and strength but also fixing the imbalances in your muscles. Now most of us have areas of our bodies that are tighter on one side than the other. This is usually our "dominant side," the side you use the most. If you are right-handed it's your right side; I'm a lefty, so my left side is always a little tighter.

Most of us have had lower back issues at some point in our lives. Sometimes these issues can be a direct result of tightness in other areas of your body, such as the hips or shoulders. If your lower back is chronically hurting (that is, it hurts all the time), then see a doctor. Some doctors specialize in the back, such as chiropractors; others deal with pain, such as acupuncturists. Massage is also good for lower back pain. Like a massage, yoga also releases tension in your muscles. One of my students, Chris Wiehl, an actor, came to my studio because of severe lower back issues. Nothing he tried worked, and he was reluctant to try yoga because he is a "guy's guy." But he's now pain-free.

Regular yoga practice (meaning you have to do it more than once a year) will help relieve the stress and tension that causes back pain. Studies have shown that yoga is the most effective exercise for relieving back pain. However, not all yoga poses relieve back pain, so it is important to know which poses will be most helpful. I've included some of the best poses for your lower back, along with modifications to make them easier. Let's take a look at the anatomy of the lower back so we can understand how it works.

How Does the Lower Back Work?

The lumbar spine has five lumbar vertebrae, which support most of your body weight when you are standing or walking. These vertebrae make up the inward curve of the lower back. The spine consists of ring-like bones called vertebrae. The vertebrae are stacked on top of each other and form a strong column that keeps the head and body standing up. Between each vertebra is a jelly-like disk that has a tough outside edge. These disks are like cushions between the vertebrae. Muscles and tissues hold your vertebrae (spine) in the right place. Located just below the lumbar vertebrae is the sacrum, which is a fused triangle-shaped vertebra. After the sacrum is another uniquely shaped vertebra, called the coccyx or tailbone, that makes up the bottom of the spine.

Most back pain is caused by irritation of the nerves that travel from the spinal cord through the bones, making the muscles tense. Irritation can be caused by stress, activity, biomechanical problems in the spine, or a herniated disk. The most common treatment for lower back pain includes medication, such as ibuprofen, and a change in lifestyle, such as losing weight. Yoga is a great form of physical activity that can help strengthen lower back muscles. It can help prevent the occurrence and recurrence of lower back injuries, which can lead to chronic

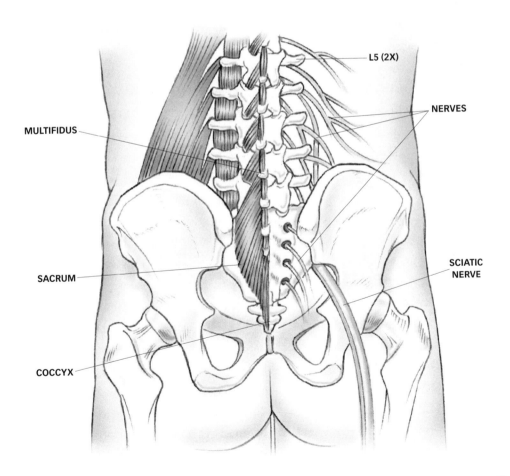

or acute pain. Yoga can strengthen your lower back muscles, make them more flexible, and alleviate pain. When it comes to the lower back, the phrase "use it or lose it" applies. The more you become a couch potato, the weaker your lower back gets. If you have a back injury, remember to contact your doctor before beginning this or any other exercise program.

Common Issues and Injuries of the Lower Back

Lower back pain: When the joints in the spine become injured or inflamed, the large back muscles can spasm. This causes lower back pain and limited range of motion. Lower back pain that lasts for more than 2 weeks can lead to muscle weakness; because using the muscles hurts, the tendency is to avoid using them. This process leads to "disuse atrophy," which means that the muscle is wasting away, and to subsequent weakening, which in turn causes more pain because the muscles are less able to help hold up the spine. It's a vicious circle. This may account for the fact that lower back pain is the second most common reason people see the doctor, topped only by colds and the flu. Sometimes you get a muscle spasm in your lower back; if your back has ever gone out you know that's not fun. I truly believe there is nothing better for the lower back than yoga. Before a back "suddenly" goes out, it's been losing its strength and flexibility for awhile. It just *seems* sudden. This is a great reason to do the "Yoga for Your Lower Back" workout routine sooner than later.

Muscles and poor posture contribute to lower back pain. Muscle strength and flexibility are essential to maintaining the neutral spine position. Weak abdominal muscles cause hip flexor muscles to tighten, increasing the curve of the lower back. Poor posture results when the curve is overextended, a condition called lordosis or swayback. I have had many students who suffer from swayback—in fact, I was working with a student in class to help her correct the curve in her lower back in Warrior 2 pose. She found that doing Warrior 2 correctly was a lot harder because it took more core strength to hold the pose with a flat instead of a curved back. That's why Chapter 8, Core/Abs, is so important for people with lower back issues. Proper posture corrects muscle imbalances that can lead to lower back pain by evenly distributing weight throughout the spine.

Another factor in lower back pain is tight hamstring muscles. Tight hamstrings limit motion in the hips and increase the stress in the lower back. Yoga focuses on strengthening and stretching the hamstring muscles. If you know your lower back pain is coming from tight hamstrings, you should read Chapter 11, Legs.

Osteoporosis: This condition affects the back and can develop without symptoms. With osteoporosis, the bones are abnormally brittle and less dense, which is the result of decreased bone mass. Usually, you don't know you have osteoporosis until a fracture occurs. Osteoporosis affects more women than men because women have less bone mass, experience menopause, and live longer. Poor diet, smoking, excessive alcohol intake, and lack of exercise also put you at a higher risk for osteoporosis.

Sciatica: The diagnosis of sciatica means that there is inflammation of the sciatic nerve. The sciatic nerve is one of the largest nerves in the body. The sciatic nerve exits the lower part of the spinal cord (lumbosacral region), passes behind the hip joint, and runs down the back of the thigh. It performs two basic functions: First, it sends signals to your muscles from the brain, and second, it collects sensory information from the legs and passes this back to your brain. Conditions such as sciatica that affect the nerve will alter these normal signals to your muscles and cause weakness of these leg muscles, pain in the legs and thighs, or both. The most common cause of sciatica is a herniated spinal disk. When this happens, the normal cushion between the vertebrae of your spine ruptures. This causes the disk to push out into areas normally occupied by these nerves. The nerves are compressed, and people then experience the symptoms of pain, weakness, and numbness. Other conditions, such as piriformis syndrome (common among runners), can also cause sciatica symptoms by irritating the nerve. Sciatica may also cause numbness and tingling or pain in the sacrum, which runs down to your foot, and can be much worse than the lower back pain.

COMMON SYMPTOMS OF SCIATICA INCLUDE:
- A cramping sensation of the thigh
- Shooting pains from the buttock down the leg
- Tingling or pins-and-needles sensations in the legs and thighs
- A burning sensation in the thigh

POSES TO HELP YOUR LOWER BACK:
1. Easy Spinal Twist
2. Knees to Chest pose
3. Dead Bug pose (or Happy Baby pose)
4. Locust pose
5. Bow pose/Half-Bow pose
6. Child's pose

Easy Spinal Twist

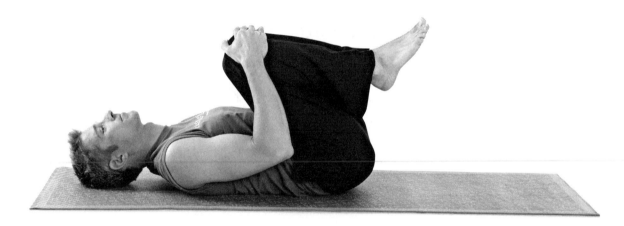

Benefits I have included Easy Spinal Twist in every workout routine. It is a great pose to gently release your lower back and can be used any time your lower back is feeling tight.

How do you get into this pose?

- Lie on the floor.
- Bring both knees to your chest.
- Hold your left knee into your chest.
- Let your right leg go straight on the floor.
- Bring your bent left knee across your body.

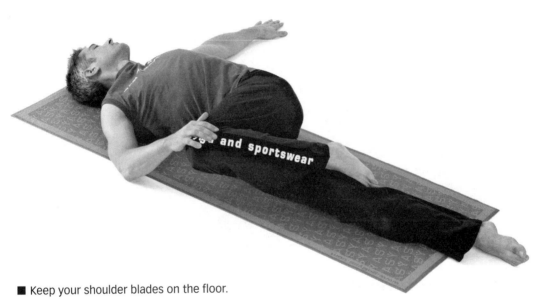

- Keep your shoulder blades on the floor.
- Look over your left shoulder to complete your twist.
- Hold for 45 seconds to 1 minute.
- Bring both knees into your chest.
- Switch sides.

Knees to Chest Pose

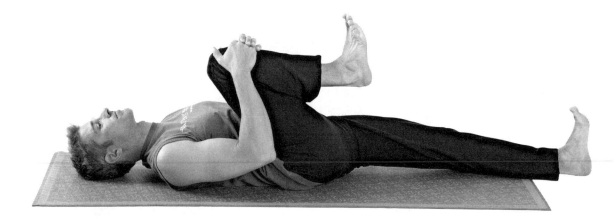

Benefits This pose stretches your lower back and relieves stiffness.

How do you get into this pose?

■ Lie flat on your back.

■ As you inhale, bend your right knee, place your hands just below the knee, and draw your leg toward your chest.

■ Your left leg should remain flat on the floor.

■ Exhale and bring your forehead up to touch your knee.

■ Inhale; as you exhale, return to your original position.

■ Repeat with the other leg.

■ Bring both knees into your chest.

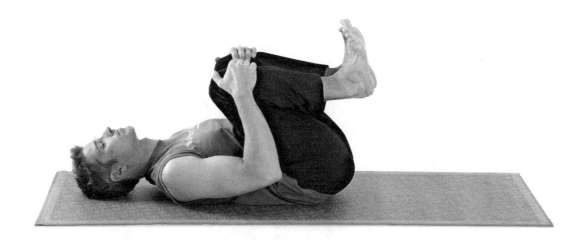

Modify the Pose Don't bring your knee in as far.

Level of Difficulty This is an easy pose. I would rate it a 5.

QUICK-FIX TIP
If you can't keep the straight leg on the floor, then bend your knee and put your foot on the floor.

Dead Bug Pose (or Happy Baby Pose)

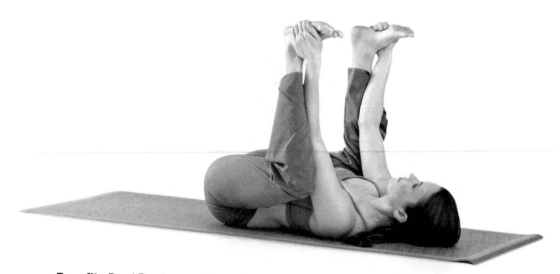

Benefits Dead Bug is a great pose for your lower back. It's one of my personal favorites. It releases your lower back but also stretches out your hips and hamstrings. This pose has been said to help sciatica, but only if you keep your lower back on the floor.

How do you get into this pose?

■ Lie down on your back.

■ Bring your knees to your chest.

■ Reach up with your hands and grab the outsides of your feet.

■ Bring your knees to the outsides of your chest.

■ Try to bring your knees toward the floor.

■ Keep your back on the floor.

■ Hold for 45 seconds to 1 minute.

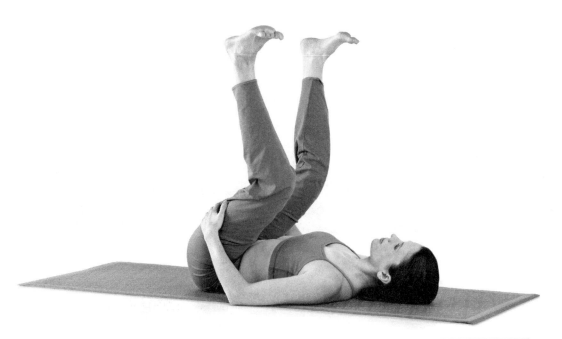

Modify the Pose If you cannot reach your feet, then grab the back of your thighs instead, and pull your thighs toward your chest.

Level of Difficulty I really like this pose—not because it's easy for me but because I like what it does for my lower back. I would rate it a solid 8.5.

QUICK-FIX TIP **Keep your spine on the floor. For this pose to be effective, your lower back needs to be on the floor. Don't worry about getting your knees to the floor; it is more important to keep your lower back flat.**

Locust Pose

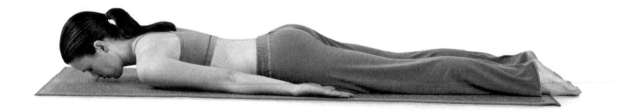

Benefits Locust strengthens the muscles in your back and in particular the lower back area. This pose isn't as easy as it looks.

How do you get into this pose?

- Lie on your stomach with your face down.
- Bring your arms alongside your body.
- Lift your head, upper body, arms, and legs up off the floor.

- Keep your arms and legs active.
- Look forward or slightly up depending on your flexibility.
- Hold for 45 seconds.
- Release everything to the floor.
- Turn your head to one side.
- Repeat three times.

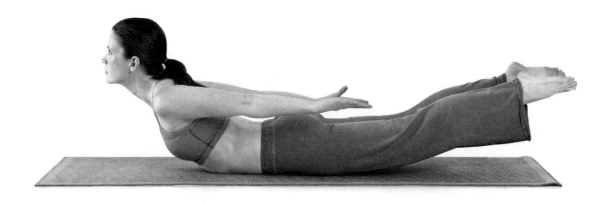

Modify the Pose You might want to try it in two parts. First, lift just the head and chest up off the floor. Then, just lift your legs off the floor while you keep the head and chest on the floor. Try to work up to lifting both the upper body and the lower body at the same time.

Level of Difficulty This pose is deceptively hard. It's one of those poses that if you just looked at the picture and never tried it, you might think, "piece of cake." Trust me, it's not easy. I'll give it a 7.5.

QUICK-FIX TIP Make sure
you are on a padded surface, like a rug, especially if you have bony hips; otherwise, this is not going to be fun.

Bow Pose (and Half-Bow Pose)

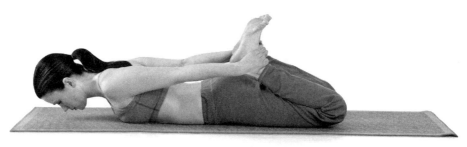

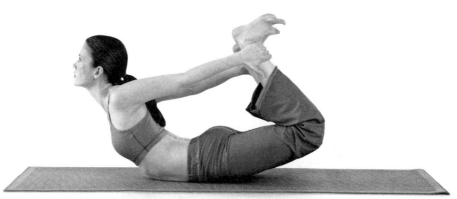

Benefits Bow opens and stretches the front of your body while strengthening your back muscles. Your back will become strong and flexible. This pose also helps improve your posture.

How do you get into this pose?

- Lie facedown on the floor.
- Bring your hands alongside your body.
- Bend your knees.
- Reach back with your hands and grab your ankles. (Don't grab your feet.)

- Keep your legs hip-distance apart.
- Lift your heels away from your body, which will pull your chest up off the floor.
- Lift your thighs and your chest off the floor.
- Keep your shoulder blades down, away from your ears.
- Hold for 30 to 45 seconds.
- Release, turning your head to the side.
- Repeat two more times.

Modify the Pose If Bow is too hard, then start with Half-Bow—just use one leg at a time. Alternatively, you can use a strap or a towel. Wrap the strap or towel around the front of your ankles.

Level of Difficulty This is not an easy pose, especially if you have tight lower back muscles. I would rate it a 9.

QUICK-FIX TIP **Make sure you are on a rug or some type of padded surface. If you have any neck issues, keep your head in a neutral position by looking down at the floor.**

Child's Pose

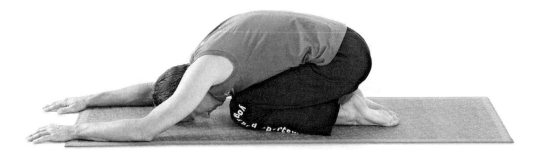

Benefits This pose is called a restorative pose or a resting pose, one you do if you get tired in a yoga class. It's an easy pose for releasing the muscles in the back. If you go to a yoga class, you will certainly do Child's pose at some point.

How do you get into this pose?

- Kneel on the floor.
- Bring your knees together.
- Rest your chest on your thighs.
- Bring your arms alongside your body.
- Let your forehead drop to the floor.
- Hold for 45 seconds to 1 minute (longer if it feels good to you).

Modify the Pose If you are having a hard time sitting on your heels, you can use a blanket. Putting the blanket on the back of your calf muscles will help prop you up.

Level of Difficulty This is a really easy pose for just about everyone, so I would rate it a 4.

QUICK-FIX TIP You can do Child's pose with your knees together. If you also want this to be a hip opener, you can spread your knees apart and rest your chest in between your thighs.

"Yoga for Your Lower Back" Workout Routine: 8 Minutes

If your back is really tight, just do the first few poses until your muscles release. You might want to take a hot bath before you do these poses so your back is warmed up.

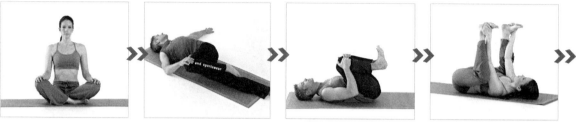

BREATH WORK

EASY SPINAL TWIST

KNEES TO CHEST POSE

DEAD BUG POSE

Come to the floor, on your mat if you have one. Sit up tall in an easy cross-legged position, and close your eyes. We are going to take a minute to center your body and get you focused on your lower back. Take a deep breath in through your nose and exhale it through your mouth. We're going to do this two more times; each time, try to hold your breath for a few moments before you exhale. Try to focus on your lower back while you are breathing.

Normally we end with this pose, but we are going to start with it because it is such a great pose to release your lower back. If you have the time to do only one of these "Yoga for Your Lower Back" poses, then do this one. Roll down onto your back, and hug your knees into your chest. Keep your left knee pressed into your chest, and let your right leg go straight on the floor. Take a deep breath in; on your next exhale, bring your left knee across your body while keeping your shoulder blades on the floor. Turn your head to the left to complete your twist. It doesn't matter how far your knee goes down toward the floor. As your back opens up and you get a little more flexible, your knee will fall closer to the floor. Hold this for about 45 seconds to 1 minute. Take a deep breath in; on your exhale, bring both knees into your chest, hug them in, and then switch sides.

Lie flat on your back. As you inhale, bend your right knee, place your hands just below the knee, and draw your leg toward your chest. Your left leg should remain flat on the floor. Exhale and bring your forehead up to touch your knee. Inhale; as you exhale, return to your original position. Hold for 30 seconds. Repeat with the other leg.

Stay lying on your back. Reach up and grab the outside of your feet and try to bring your knees down by your sides. If you cannot reach your feet, grab the backs of your thighs. This pose is great for releasing the lower back (the sacrum), but you have to make sure your lower back is on the floor. Hold for 45 seconds to 1 minute.

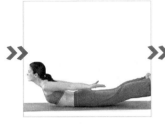

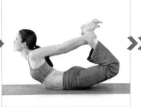

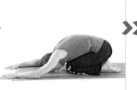

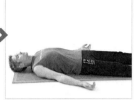

LOCUST POSE

BOW POSE

CHILD'S POSE

CORPSE POSE

From Dead Bug pose, I want you to flip onto your stomach. You want to make sure you are on a rug or a padded surface, especially if you have bony hips. Lie face-down with arms at the sides, palms down, your elbows slightly bent, and your fingers pointing toward your feet. Raise your legs and thighs as high off the ground as possible without causing your back any pain. Hold for 10 seconds and repeat three times. This can be a hard pose, so make sure you don't strain already injured muscles. Then release everything back to the floor, turn your head to one side, and just rest for a few seconds. Repeat two more times. If you have any neck issues, keep your neck flat by looking at the ground.

This can be a very challenging pose. You can modify it if you want by either using a strap or a towel or by doing Half-Bow. Stay on your stomach, bend your knees, and bring the soles of your feet to the ceiling. Reach back with your hands and grab your ankles. If you can't reach your ankles, use a strap or towel to help you; wrap the strap around the front of your ankles. Take a deep breath in and on your exhale pull your feet away from your body. This will lift your chest off the floor. Repeat this one more time.

Kneel on the floor. Bring your knees together. Rest your chest on your thighs. Bring your arms alongside your body. Let your forehead drop to the floor. Hold for 45 seconds to 1 minute.

Lie on your back. Put a blanket under your knees, or keep your knees bent in this pose instead of having your legs straight out on the floor. This relieves any tension in your lower back. Close your eyes. Take a deep breath in and on your exhale, just let your whole body sink into the floor. Corpse pose helps the body adjust to what you just did; it allows the benefits of your yoga workout routine to sink into your body, before you run off. Let your whole body relax, making sure you focus on your lower back. Stay here for about 2 minutes to get the maximum benefits. After you are completely relaxed, take a deep breath in through your nose and just "sigh" it out. Bend your knees, roll onto your right side for a few seconds, then push yourself up to a comfortable, easy, cross-legged position like we started with. Bring your hands together in front of your chest, take a deep breath in, and on your exhale bow forward. Take a second to appreciate the fact that you did something good for yourself today.

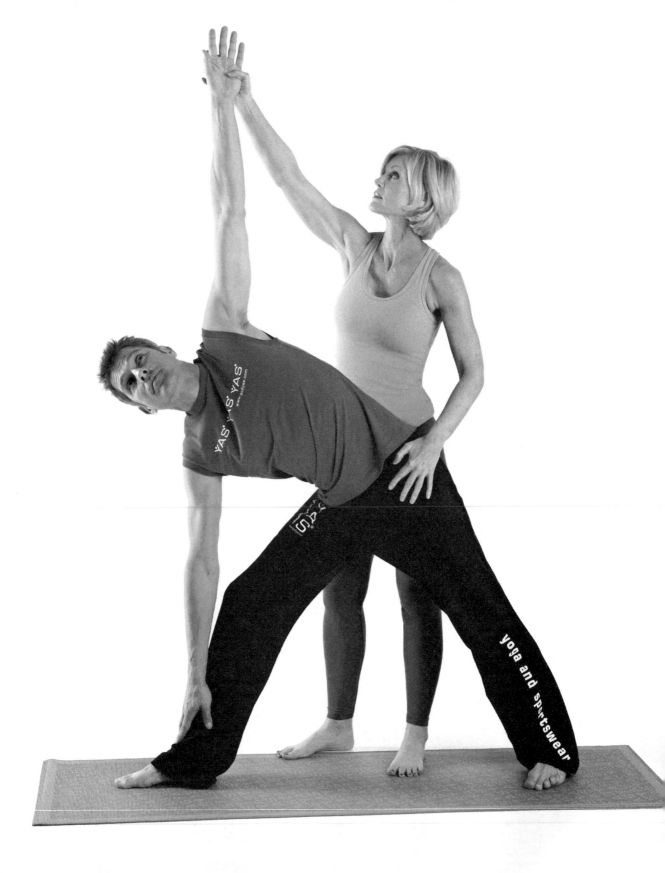

chapter 10

Hips

Hip Hip Hooray

When you are young, your hips are very flexible—they have wide range of motion. If you don't believe me, watch a 4-year-old walk. As we age, our bodies start to round forward. Our hips get tight, our shoulders round forward, and we lose that mobility (flexibility) that we had when we were young. The yoga poses in the "Yoga for Your Hips" workout routine will help restore mobility in your hips. But I'm not promising that you will run around like a 4-year-old!

I have always found the hips fascinating. When you think about it, you realize that without them we can't do much of anything. Almost all poses in yoga work on your hips in one way or another; that's how important hips are to the overall function and health of your body. I am going to talk about the anatomy of the hips, but don't worry. There's nothing too complicated—I just want to give you an idea of how they work so you have a better understanding of the ways yoga can help prevent injury and improve all-around body mechanics of your hip joints and the muscles around the hip.

How Do the Hips Work?

The hip is the most stable joint in the body, and it is surrounded by muscle on all sides. The multiple muscles attach to the back, abdomen, hamstrings, quadriceps, abductors, adductors, and gluteal muscles; this gives the hips great range of motion. Most muscles of the hip are shorter and fatter than those of the leg. They allow rotation, which helps stabilize the hip joint. Most hip injuries occur when these small muscles are overused or pushed too hard.

The hip is a ball-and-socket joint in which the head of the femur (the thigh bone) meets the pelvic bone. The pelvic bone fits tightly around the head of the femur. The ball is held in the socket by very powerful ligaments (the joint capsule) that form a complete sleeve around the joint. The capsule has a thin lining called the synovial fluid. The head of the femur is covered with a layer of smooth cartilage. The socket is also lined with cartilage. This cartilage cushions the joint and allows the bones to move on each other with very little friction.

The hip joint itself is capable of a wide range of motion because the joint is supported by four sets of muscles and connecting tendons that operate together with machine-like precision. The hip flexors, extensors, adductors, and external rotators combine to provide a 360-degree range of motion. The importance of the hip joint is not only the range of motion that it allows the upper leg but also the considerable muscular power and endurance that is delivered in concert with the motion.

The hip joint flexor supports the process of flexion (the movement of the hip joint that produces a bend), which helps propel the legs forward and upward. Extension is the hip action that straightens the leg. Through rotation, the hip joint directs the femur and the upper thigh through the 360-degree range of motion. Adduction is movement of the hip

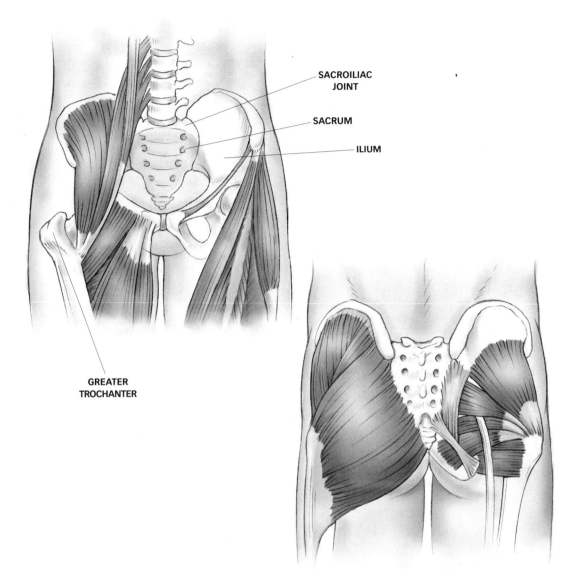

SACROILIAC
JOINT

SACRUM

ILIUM

GREATER
TROCHANTER

muscles that draws the femur and upper thigh toward the body; the adductors are important stabilizing muscles in running.

There are also a lot of ligaments in the hip joint that connect the femur to the pelvis. They are responsible for stabilizing the hip. These ligaments prevent the hip from moving outside the possible planes of movements. Muscles play an important part in stabilizing the lower part of your body and are powerhouses for the hip in locomotion activities. The muscles are involved when the limbs are raised or lowered. Overdeveloped and tight hip flexors can contribute to lower back pain by causing the pelvis to tilt forward. To counteract this, you must stretch the hip flexors and strengthen the abdominal muscles (which we talked about in the core/abs chapter). This will reduce pelvic tilt and decrease lower back pain. Strengthening the lower back can also help improve the balance between the muscles of the hip region.

Common Injuries of the Hips

Hip bursitis: This common problem causes pain over the outside of the upper thigh. A bursa is a fluid-filled sac that allows smooth motion between two uneven surfaces. For example, in the hip, a bursa rests between the bony prominence over the outside of the hip (the greater trochanter) and the firm tendon that passes over this bone. When the bursal sac becomes inflamed, pain occurs each time the tendon has to move over the bone. Because people with hip bursitis move this tendon with each step, hip bursitis can be quite painful; the condition is commonly seen in runners or athletes who participate in running-oriented sports, such as soccer, football, and basketball.

Broken hip: A broken hip is a common injury, especially as we get older. In the United States, hip fractures are the most common broken bone—about 300,000 Americans are hospitalized for a hip fracture every year. Hip fractures in the elderly are most often caused by a fall, usually a seemingly insignificant fall. In younger patients with stronger bones, more common causes of a broken hip include high-energy injuries such as car accidents.

Snapping-hip syndrome: Snapping-hip syndrome is characterized by a snapping sensation, and often an audible popping noise, when the hip is flexed and extended. It most commonly results from tendons catching on bony prominences and "snapping" when the hip is moved. There are three primary causes:

■ **Iliotibial band snap:** The iliotibial band (the IT band) is a thick, wide tendon that runs over the outside of the hip joint. The most common cause of snapping-hip syndrome is snapping of the iliotibial band over the greater trochanter (what you think of as the hipbone). If this is causing your snapping-hip syndrome, you may develop trochanteric bursitis from the irritation of the bursa in that area.

- ■ **Iliopsoas tendon snap:** The iliopsoas tendon is the main hip flexor muscle, and the tendon of this muscle passes just in front of the hip joint. The iliopsoas tendon can catch on a bony part of the pelvis (what you think of as your hip bone), causing a snap when the hip is flexed. Usually, people with iliopsoas tendon as the cause of snapping-hip syndrome have no problems, but they may find the snapping annoying.

- ■ **Hip labral tear:** The least common cause of snapping-hip syndrome is a tear of the cartilage within the hip joint. If a loose flap of cartilage is catching within the joint, a snapping sensation (sometimes with a "pop") may occur when the hip is moved. A hip labral tear may also cause an unsteady feeling, and people will grab for support when the hip snaps.

Iliotibial band syndrome: This syndrome is due to inflammation of the iliotibial band, a thick band of fibrous tissue that runs down the outside of the leg. The iliotibial band begins at the hip and extends to the outer side of the shinbone (tibia) just below the knee joint. The band functions in coordination with several of the thigh muscles to provide stability to the outside of the knee joint.

POSES TO HELP YOUR HIPS:

1. Leg Cradle pose
2. Foot to Knee pose (aka Seated Tree pose)
3. Cobbler pose
4. Happy Cow pose
5. Reclining Pigeon pose

Leg Cradle Pose

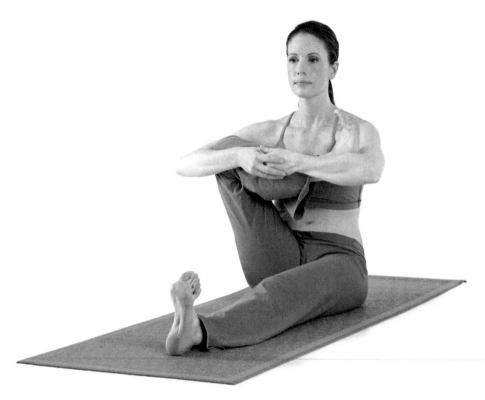

Benefits This pose loosens up your hip joint. I always do this pose before I run.

How do you get into this pose?

■ Sit on the floor with both legs out in front of you.

QUICK-FIX TIP **Sit with your back up against the wall.**

■ Grab your right leg and "cradle" it in your arms—your foot should be in the crease of your left arm and your knee should be in the crease of your right arm.

■ Rock it side to side for 30 seconds.

■ Switch sides.

Modify the Pose Don't pull your shin to your chest; just go to your level of flexibility.

Level of Difficulty This is an easy pose. I'll give it a 5.

Foot to Knee Pose (aka Seated Tree Pose)

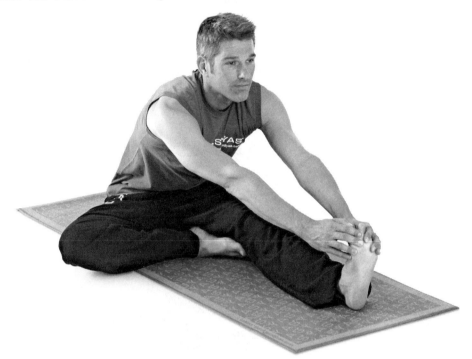

Benefits This pose opens your hip in an outward rotation. We are going to work on stretching and opening every muscle around the hip joint.

How do you get into this pose?

■ Sit on the floor with your legs together and straight out in front of you.

■ Bring the sole of your right foot to the inside of your left knee. If that's uncomfortable, then bring your foot down your leg to your calf.

■ Sit up straight; make sure your hips are square (not leaning to one side or the other).

■ Reach your arms up to the ceiling.

■ Hinge at your hips and try to reach your toes.

■ Try to grab your foot. If you can't reach your foot, then use a strap or a towel to help out.

■ Hold for 45 seconds to 1 minute.

Modify the Pose Bring your foot down to your calf; you can also sit up on a blanket.

Level of Difficulty This is a fairly easy pose—I'll give it a 5.5.

QUICK-FIX TIP **The more flexible you are, the higher up the thigh your foot will go. So as you work on this pose and your hips open up, try to bring your foot closer to your upper thigh and groin area.**

Knee to Ankle Pose (aka Fire Log Pose)

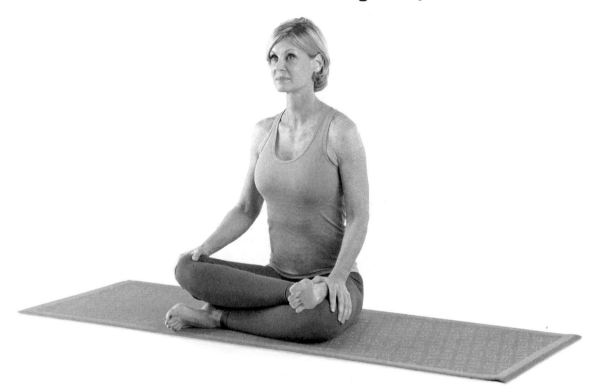

Benefits This pose stretches your hips and your groin area.

How do you get into this pose?

- Come down to the floor in a seated position.
- Bend your legs and put your right leg on top of your left leg.
- Bring your right ankle to the outside of your left knee.
- Flex both of your feet.
- Sit up tall.

- Hold for 45 seconds to 1 minute.
- Switch sides.

Modify the Pose To make this pose more challenging, lean forward from your hips.

Level of Difficulty I don't know about you, but I find this pose hard. I would rate it a 7.

QUICK-FIX TIP **If you have really tight hips, try sitting up on a blanket.**

Cobbler Pose

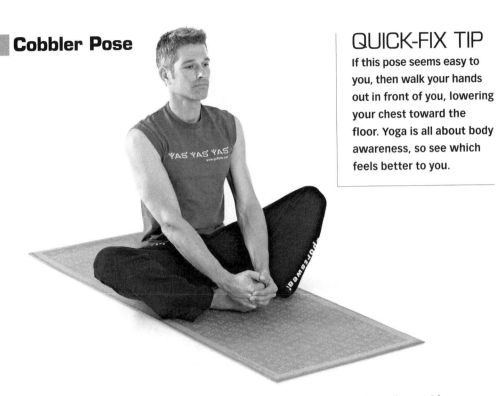

QUICK-FIX TIP

If this pose seems easy to you, then walk your hands out in front of you, lowering your chest toward the floor. Yoga is all about body awareness, so see which feels better to you.

Benefits This pose opens and stretches not only your hips but also your lower back and your inner thighs. All of these muscles work together to keep your hips working. The sports that benefit from this pose include running, cycling, soccer, hockey, skiing (on both snow and water), football, and basketball. This pose is helpful for sports injuries such as piriformis syndrome, groin strain, tendonitis of the adductor muscles, and hip bursitis.

How do you get into this pose?

- Sit on the floor with your legs out in front of you.
- Bring the soles of your feet together and your knees wide apart.
- Bring the heels of your feet toward your body.
- Sit up straight, grab your feet for leverage, take a deep breath in, and

on your exhale hinge forward from your hips.

- Keep your back straight to get the maximum benefit from this pose.
- Don't force yourself down in this pose; focus on keeping your back straight. Whether your nose is hitting the ground or you can lean forward only a few inches, you are still getting the benefit from this pose.

Modify the Pose If you find that your knees are way up in the air, then you can move your feet away from your body or use your elbows to push your knees down, whichever works for you.

Level of Difficulty For most athletes, and guys in general, this is a tough pose. I would rate it a 7.5.

Happy Cow Pose (aka Cow Face Pose)

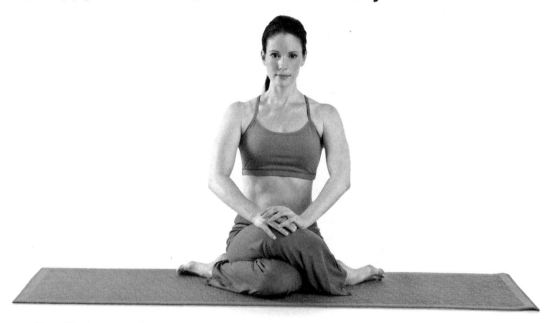

Benefits I never understood why this pose was called Happy Cow. Once you get into the pose, do you look like a cow? Regardless of the name, it's a great pose for stretching and opening your hips, as well as your thighs, shoulders, triceps, and chest.

How do you get into this pose?

- Sit on the floor with both legs out in front of you.
- Bring your right leg on top of your left leg.
- Bring both of your feet toward your body.

QUICK-FIX TIPS Use a strap to help you with the arm part of this pose. Hold the strap with the top arm and let it fall down your back so you can grab it with the bottom arm. If your hips are really tight, then sit up on a blanket.

- Line your knees on top of each other.
- Sit up tall.
- Bring your right arm up in the air.
- Bend your right arm at the elbow and drop it behind your back.
- Bring your left arm behind your back.
- Try to clasp your hands together.
- Hold for 45 seconds to 1 minute.
- Release your legs and arms and switch sides.

Modify the Pose If the arm part of this pose is too hard to do, you can skip it for now because this workout is for your hips. If you want more of a challenge, you can lean forward in this pose, bringing your upper body toward the floor. But I think this pose is hard enough, just on its own!

Level of Difficulty This pose is hard to do; I would rate it a 7.5.

Reclining Pigeon Pose

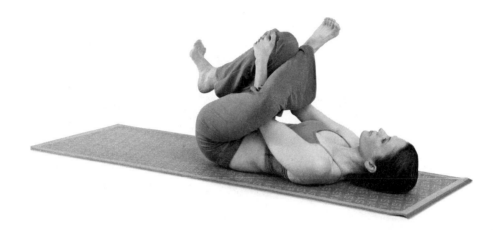

Benefits This pose helps open the hip area by stretching the muscles around the hip joint. You should feel a great stretch in the muscles around your hip. If you have time to do only one hip-opener pose, this would be the one I suggest doing.

How do you get into this pose?

- Start by lying down on your back.
- Bend your knees with your feet on the floor about hip-distance apart.
- Bring your left foot up and place it on top of your right thigh; your ankle should hit just below the knee of the bent right leg.
- Take your left arm and reach it through your legs.
- Take your right arm and bring it on the outside of your right leg.
- Try to grab your shin with both hands, lacing your fingers together.
- Gently pull your shin toward your chest, but

only go to the point where you can keep your head and shoulders on the ground.
- Hold this pose for 1 minute and then work up to 3 minutes.
- Switch sides.

Modify the Pose Grab the back of your leg instead until your hip releases. Then try to grab onto your shin.

Level of Difficulty This pose is an easier version of Full Pigeon, but for most of us with tight hips it is still a hard pose. I would rate it a 6.5.

QUICK-FIX TIP **Don't force this pose; stay relaxed to get the maximum benefit. Because there are so many muscles around the hip joint, this is a pose you need to hold for a while.**

"Yoga for Your Hips" Workout Routine: 10 Minutes

This routine is safe to do whether you are warmed up or not, but I would prefer you be warmed up to get the maximum benefit out of the poses. If you are participating in a sport, then try to do "Yoga for Your Hips" after your workout.

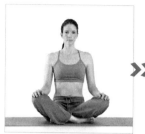 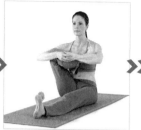 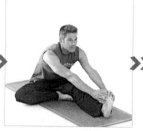 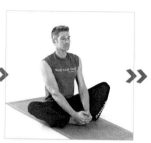

BREATH WORK

LEG CRADLE POSE

FOOT TO KNEE POSE

COBBLER POSE

Come to the floor, on your mat if you have one. Sit up tall in an easy cross-legged pose and close your eyes. We are going to take a minute to center your body and get you focused on your hips. Take a deep breath in through your nose and exhale it through your mouth. Repeat two more times; each time try to hold your breath for a few moments before you exhale.

Stay seated on the floor with both legs out in front of you. Grab your right leg and "cradle" it in your arms so that your foot is in the crease of your left arm and your knee is in the crease of your right arm. Rock it side to side for 30 seconds, then switch sides.

Stay seated on the floor with your legs together and straight out in front of you. Bring the sole of your right foot to the inside of your left knee. Sit up tall, making sure you keep your hips squared. Take a deep breath in and on your exhale hinge forward. Try to reach your foot—if you can't, use a towel.

From here bring the soles of your feet together and your knees wide apart. Bring the heels of your feet toward your body. Sit up straight, grab your feet for leverage, take a deep breath in, and on your exhale hinge forward from your hips. Try to keep your back straight to get the maximum benefit from this pose. Don't force yourself down in this pose; focus on keeping your back straight. Whether your nose is hitting the ground or you can lean forward only a few inches, you are still getting the benefit from this pose.

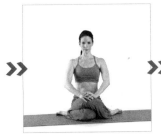

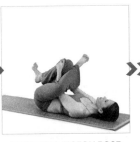

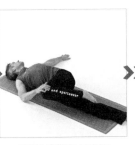

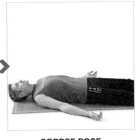

HAPPY COW POSE

RECLINING PIGEON POSE

EASY SPINAL TWIST

CORPSE POSE

Sit on the floor with both legs out in front of you. Bring your right leg on top of your left leg. Bring both of your feet toward your body and make sure you line up your knees on top of each other. Sit up tall. From here we are going to add the arm part of this pose, so bring your right arm up in the air. Bend your right arm at the elbow and drop it behind your back. Bring your left arm behind your back. Try to clasp your hands together. Hold for 45 seconds to 1 minute. Release your legs and arms and switch sides.

Stay seated, but roll down onto your back. Bend your knees with your feet on the floor about hip-distance apart. Bring your left foot up and place it on top of your right leg; your ankle should hit just below the knee of the bent right leg. The knee of the left leg is bent out to the side—it should look like a triangle. Now take your left arm and reach it through your legs; take your right arm and bring it on the outside of your right leg. Try to grab your shin with both hands, lacing your fingers together. Now pull your shin toward your chest, but go only to the point where you can keep your head and shoulders on the ground. You should feel a great stretch in the muscles around your hip. Hold this pose for 1 minute and then work up to 3 minutes. Switch sides. It is very common to have one side of your body tighter than the other. Our goal in yoga in general is to balance out the body. With this pose in particular you might notice the imbalances in your hips. Hold this pose for 1 minute and work up to 3 minutes.

Come down to the floor on your back and then hug your knees into your chest. Bring your left knee into your chest and keep your right leg straight on the floor. Bring your left knee across your body while keeping your shoulder blades on the floor. Look over your left shoulder to complete this twist. Hold for 20 to 30 seconds, then hug both knees into your chest. Switch sides. The right knee comes into your chest, and the left leg goes straight. Bring the right knee across your body and look over your right shoulder to complete the twist on the right side. Take a second to notice the difference from one side to the other. Hold for 20 to 30 seconds, then bring both knees into your chest.

From here we are going into our final pose, Corpse pose. Lie down on your back, and bring your arms out by your sides. Close your eyes; if you want to, you can put a towel over your eyes to help you relax. Take a deep breath in and on your exhale just let your whole body sink into the floor. We are going to end this workout like we started it, with a little breath work. Remember, don't skip this part; it helps the body adjust to what you just did. It allows the benefits of your workout routine to sink into your body before you run off. Let your whole body relax, and make sure you focus on your hips. Notice whether there is any tightness in your body, and then relax that area. Stay here for about 2 minutes to get the maximum benefits. Bend your knees, roll onto your right side for a few seconds, then push yourself up to a comfortable, easy, cross-legged position like we started with. Take a second to appreciate the fact that you did something good for yourself today. Your hips will definitely thank you!

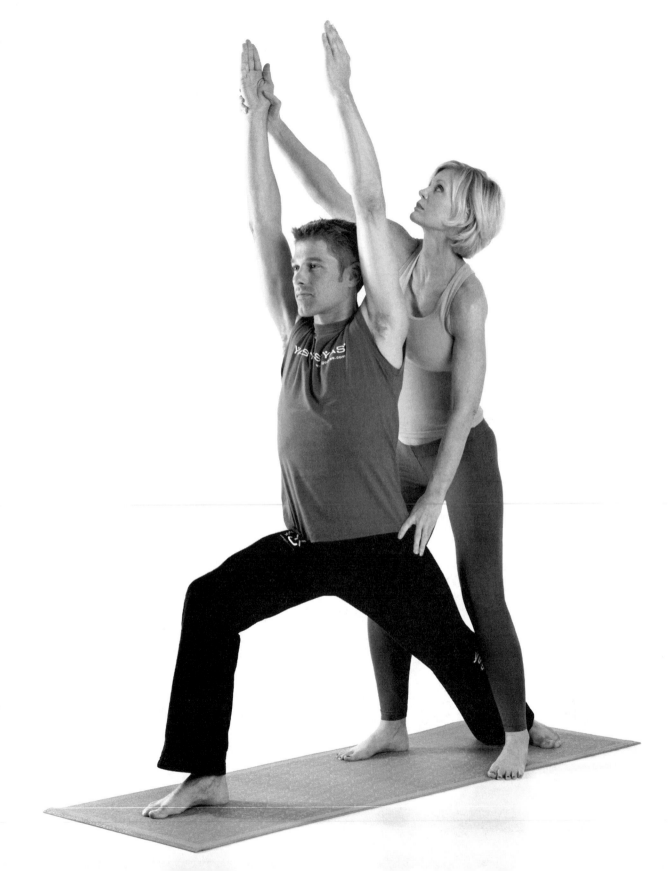

chapter 11

Legs

Divided We Stand

We are going to focus on the main muscles in your legs: the quadriceps, hamstrings, and calf muscles. Your hamstrings have two main actions: flexion, which is what happens when you bend your knees, and extension of your knees and hips, which is what happens when you are down on the ground and go to stand up. Just about every "standing pose" in yoga works some part of, if not all of, your legs. I'm going to show you how yoga not only can help build strength and flexibility in your legs but also help prevent and/or heal common injuries, such as shin splints. If you are a runner, I'm sure you have dealt with shin splints or a torn calf muscle. Unfortunately for me, since I am a major runner, I experienced most of these injuries before I really got into yoga. In fact, I remember popping my hamstring right before my first marathon.

I had been training like crazy. My legs were so tight I could barely walk, but I could still run. I know some of you who are runners are laughing right now because you know what I'm talking about. I saw a bar where some people were stretching and I thought, "Hmmm, I should probably stretch. I heard it's good for tight muscles." I flung my leg up on a 4-foot-high bar, and guess what happened? You got it—I popped my hamstring! I was on the ground, so pissed off; I had trained so hard! I swore at that moment, "I will never stretch again." It was one of those moments where I can look back and apply the saying "If you want to make God laugh, tell him your plans." Now all these years later, I'm a yoga expert? Unbelievable!

Now, as I have told you, some chapters are easier than others. This one is going to be challenging. When it comes to using your leg muscles in yoga, it means doing what are called "standing poses." I am sure you have heard of poses called Warrior 1 and Warrior 2, right? These are basic poses in most yoga classes, especially power yoga, which links poses to build heat in your body.

How Do the Legs Work?

The muscles and joints of the legs provide strength and stability for the body, which allows us to use our body weight for such activities as walking, running, and jumping. Basically, if we want to move, we need to use our legs. Several muscles in the legs are considered the largest muscle groups in the body. So what are the main muscles in the legs?

Quadriceps and hamstrings are what we normally think of. The quadriceps, composed of four muscles that cover the front of the thigh, straighten the leg at the knee. The hamstring muscles are actually a group of three muscles that run down the back part of the upper leg. Together, this group of muscles—the biceps femoris, the semitendinosus, and the semimembranosus—bend the leg at the knee and extend the leg at the hip joint. This action allows us to run, walk, and jump. All muscles work in pairs to perform a task. One set of muscles shortens to exert force, while the other set of muscles relaxes. The hamstring muscles, located at the back of the thigh, work with the quadriceps muscles in the front of the thigh. When you bend your leg, the hamstring muscles contract and the quadriceps muscles relax. Conversely, when you straighten your leg, the quadriceps muscles contract and the hamstring muscles relax.

The other two large muscles in the legs are the gluteus maximus and the sartorius. The former is a large, wide muscle that covers the back of the hip joint and comprises your butt. It extends and rotates the leg. The sartorius, the longest muscle in the body, runs

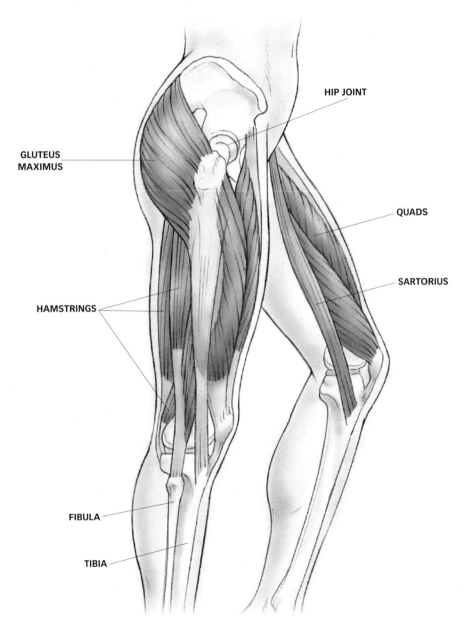

from the hipbone diagonally across the front of the thigh to the inside of the knee, and bends the leg at both the hip and the knee.

Your legs, hips, knees, and feet all work together to allow your legs to move. The upper part of your leg, the thigh, is supported by the femur—the longest and strongest bone of the body. The upper end of the femur is rounded and fits into a cavity in the hipbone, forming a ball-and-socket joint, which we talked about in Chapter 10. The ball-and-socket joint of the hip permits circular motion and allows your leg to move in almost any direction. This joint also helps distribute body weight evenly over the head of the femur. At the knee, the femur connects to the tibia, or shinbone, to form a hinge joint. Hinge joints permit back-and-forth movement similar to the motion of a hinged door. This joint is protected in front by a small triangular bone called the patella, or kneecap, which lies in the tendon covering the joint.

The tibia is one of the two long bones of the lower leg. It forms the front of the leg; the fibula, which is somewhat smaller, forms the side of the leg. The upper end of the fibula joins the tibia just below the knee joint. The tibia and fibula connect to the talus, or anklebone, at the ankle joint, which is a hinged joint.

Common Injuries of the Legs and How to Prevent and Treat Them

Hamstring injury: A hamstring injury (aka posterior femoral muscle strain) is any injury to the hamstring muscles. Hamstring injuries can occur when the leg is suddenly extended fully, such as with kicking a ball or doing a kick in kickboxing. Or, as in my case, throwing your leg up on a bar! Sprinting is another very common cause; for example, sprinting suddenly without warming up your legs or sprinting after a hard training session the day before can injure the hamstrings. A direct blow from a hockey stick or racket can also do the damage; this happened to one of my students the other day—ouch!

What is a pulled hamstring? Anyone who watches sports knows that a pulled hamstring is a troublesome and sometimes painful condition for athletes. Pulled hamstrings typically occur when the knee extends and the muscle is contracted suddenly. Pulled hamstring muscles are a common sports-related injury and can be a result of insufficient warmup.

TYPES OF HAMSTRING TEARS

■ Grade 1 tear: The muscle is tender but not bruised.

■ Grade 2 tear: Bruising is seen where the muscle fibers tore.

■ Grade 3 tear: Bruising and actual separation of the muscle occur.

TREATING A PULLED OR TORN HAMSTRING

Rest and application of ice to the affected area are required for proper healing. After healing begins, exercises like the "Yoga for Your Legs" workout can be used to strengthen the hamstrings and help prevent recurrent injury.

Anyone can experience hamstring strain, but people at risk for this injury are:

■ Adolescent athletes who are still growing

■ Professional athletes (football or soccer players, skaters)

■ Runners or sprinters

■ Dancers

Hamstring injuries are easier to prevent than to cure, which is why it is good to start doing yoga. The best way to prevent a hamstring injury is to do yoga before an activity so your hamstrings are warmed up. Weak or tight hamstrings can contribute to lower back pain, so doing the "Yoga for Your Legs" workout routine to strengthen and stretch the hamstrings may also reduce your risk for lower back pain.

Strains and tears: When one muscle group is much stronger than its opposing muscle group, the imbalance can lead to a strain. This frequently happens with the hamstring muscles. The quadriceps muscles are usually much more powerful, so the hamstring may become fatigued faster than the quadriceps. A fatigued muscle cannot relax as easily when its opposing muscle contracts, leading to strains.

Muscle strains are overuse injuries that result when the muscle is stretched without being properly warmed up. It's like pulling a rubber band too far. Eventually, the rubber band will either lose its shape or tear apart. The same thing happens with muscles. Hamstring injuries are usually easy to spot.

■ Mild strains may involve a simple tightening of the muscle that you can feel.

■ More severe injuries may result in a sharp pain in the back of the thigh.

■ A rupture or tear may leave you unable to stand or walk. The muscle may be tender to the touch, and it may be painful to stretch your leg. Within a few days after a tear, bruising may appear.

Shin splints: A shin splint is pain resulting from damage to the muscles along the shin (the area between the front of your knee and your ankle). Shin splints may develop in the muscles in the front and outer parts of the shin. Pain is felt in different areas, depending on which muscles are affected. The usual cause is repeated stress to the lower leg from activities such as running.

Calf strain or tear: Calf strain, or calf muscle strain, is a tear or a partial tear of the calf muscles. The damage can be anywhere within the muscle or tendon. A torn calf muscle occurs when part of your lower leg muscle is pulled from your Achilles tendon. It causes a sharp burning sensation, and you will usually see a bruise almost immediately from the tear of the muscle and the blood pooling in the area. I tore my calf muscles recently—it's painful! While you are recovering, you will have to modify the "Yoga for Your Legs" poses.

Thigh muscle strain: The thigh has four linked muscles at the front, which are the quadriceps group, and they join up at the kneecap. These muscles control your legs all the time that you are using them; for example, it may be obvious that the muscles work hard while you are running up a hill, but they work harder when you are running down a hill because they are controlling the knee movements at speed. They also constantly work to keep the body balanced. Thigh muscle strain can occur from overuse, and the muscle damage is not usually severe. A full or complete tear is often caused by a direct blow, as in football during a tackle. A partial tear usually results from sudden twisting or stopping movements. An overuse injury develops from repetitive activity, such as long-distance running or practice sessions consisting of constantly kicking a ball or practicing a shot in racket sports.

POSES TO HELP YOUR LEGS:

1. Warrior 1 pose

2. Warrior 2 pose

3. Triangle pose

4. Half Moon pose

5. Crescent Lunge pose

6. Legs Up a Wall pose

Warrior 1 Pose

QUICK-FIX TIP

Your "goal" in this pose is to get your thigh parallel to the floor, but make sure you keep your knee in line with your ankle.

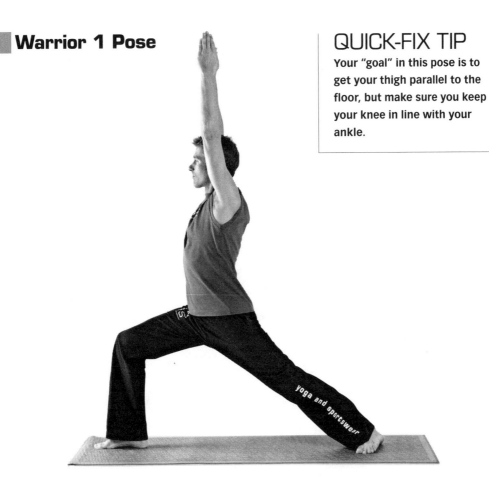

Benefits This pose strengthens all the muscles in your legs and increases the flexibility in your hips.

How do you get into this pose?

- Come to a standing position.
- Bring your legs about 3 to 4 feet apart; depending on your height, it may be a shorter or farther distance.
- Turn your right foot out so it is facing the front of the room and turn your left foot slightly in.
- Bend your knee to a 90-degree angle.

- Bring your arms to the ceiling, with your palms facing each other.
- Hold for 45 seconds to 1 minute.
- Switch sides.

Modify the Pose Don't bend your knee so much.

Level of Difficulty Standing poses can be challenging; they use most of the muscles in your body. If you just stood in Warrior 1 for 5 minutes, you would be drenched with sweat, so I would give this pose a 7.5.

Warrior 2 Pose

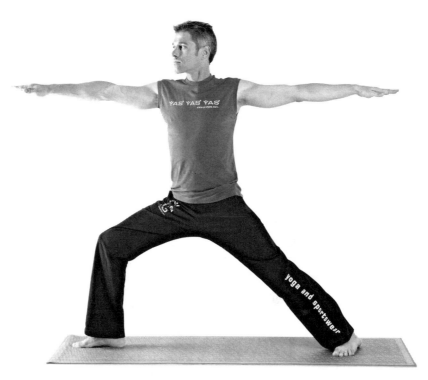

Benefits This pose strengthens and stretches the legs, ankles, and feet. When it is part of a "flow" routine, it increases your stamina.

How do you get into this pose?

■ Stand up.

■ Step your feet about 3 to 4 feet apart.

■ Raise your arms to shoulder level, palms down.

■ Turn your right foot out; it should be straight out in front of you.

■ Turn your left foot in slightly.

■ Bend your front knee; eventually you want the thigh parallel to the floor, but for now just go down as far as you can.

■ Make sure your back leg is straight and strong.

■ Hold for 30 seconds to 1 minute.

■ Switch sides.

Modify the Pose Don't go down as far in the pose.

Level of Difficulty All Warrior poses are meant to be strong poses, hence the name "Warrior." I had to hold this pose for about 10 minutes for a photo shoot; I truly thought I was going to die. So I would give it a solid 8.

QUICK-FIX TIP **Make sure your knee stays in line with your ankle.**

Triangle Pose

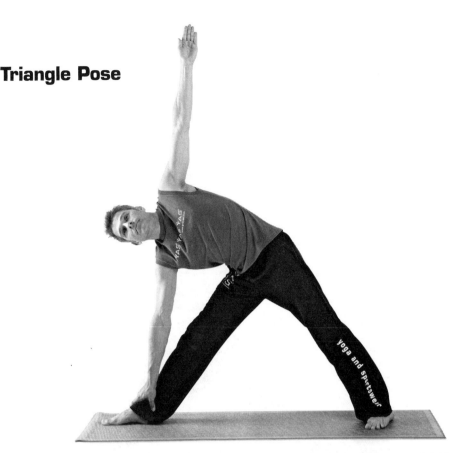

Benefits Triangle pose has a lot of benefits for your leg muscles; it stretches and strengthens your thighs, knees, and ankles. It also stretches your inner thigh, hamstrings, and calves. It is a basic pose in most yoga classes, so you may have already heard of it. Triangle, like most poses in yoga, works many areas of your body. It improves the strength and stability of your legs and feet while opening your upper body.

How do you get into this pose?

- From a standing position, step your feet about 3 to 4 feet apart.
- Keep your legs straight.
- Turn your right foot straight out in front of you and turn your left foot slightly inward.
- Bring your arms out to your sides, like a T.
- Lean forward and bring your right hand to your shin.
- Bring your left hand to the ceiling.
- Look straight ahead or to the ceiling, depending on the flexibility of your neck.
- Hold for 30 seconds to 1 minute.
- Switch sides.
- Keep your left foot straight out and turn your right foot in slightly.

Level of Difficulty This is an easy pose, so I would give it a 5.5.

QUICK-FIX TIP Try to keep your body straight—don't let your butt stick out.

Crescent Lunge Pose

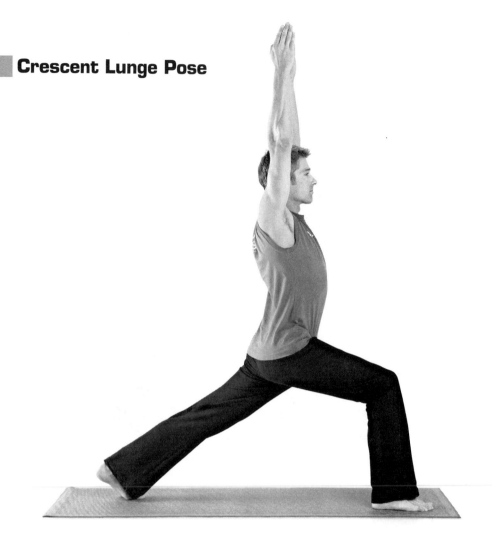

Benefits This pose strengthens your legs and stretches your hips.

How do you get into this pose?

- From Half Moon, move back through Warrior 2, shifting your weight onto the ball of your back foot and bringing your hands to your hips.
- Stay up on the ball of your back foot.
- Lift your upper body so you are standing up straight.
- Keep your hips squared.
- Bring your arms above you and reach for the ceiling. Palms should be facing each other.
- Hold for 30 seconds to 1 minute.
- Switch sides.

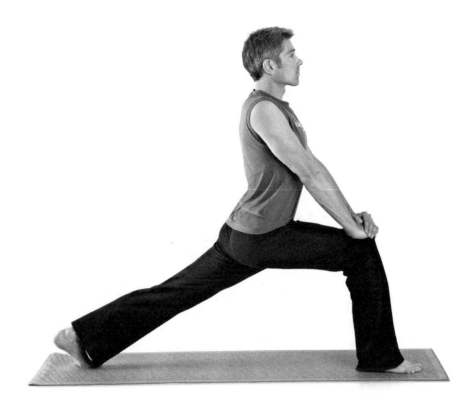

Modify the Pose Instead of staying up on the ball of your back foot, drop your knee to the floor. You might know this as a "runners lunge."

Level of Difficulty This is a hard pose to hold; I would rate it a 7.5.

QUICK-FIX TIP I want you to notice whether one side is tighter than the other. You will probably feel a difference in your hip flexors. One of the goals of this pose is to balance out your hips, and if you do this routine two or three times a week you will definitely start to undo any imbalances in your legs.

■ Half Moon Pose

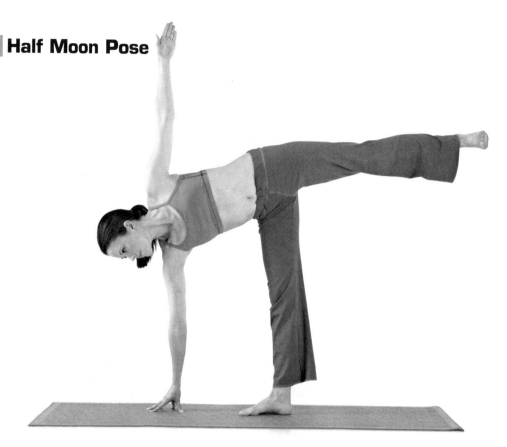

Benefits This pose strengthens your legs and stretches your hips, hamstrings, and inner thighs.

How do you get into this pose?

- Start from Triangle with your right leg in front.
- Bring your right hand to the floor about a foot in front of you.

QUICK-FIX TIP **Try to stack your hips on top of each other, and don't lean on your bottom arm. Let core strength hold you up in this pose. Remember to breathe!**

- Bring your left leg up to hip level and flex your foot.
- Bring your left arm up to the ceiling.
- Hold for 45 seconds to 1 minute.
- Switch sides.

Modify the Pose If you find it hard to reach your hand to the floor and keep your back straight, use a block or several books to rest your hand on.

Level of Difficulty This is an easy balancing pose, but it's still a balancing pose so there is a degree of difficulty. I would rate it a 6.5.

Legs Up a Wall Pose

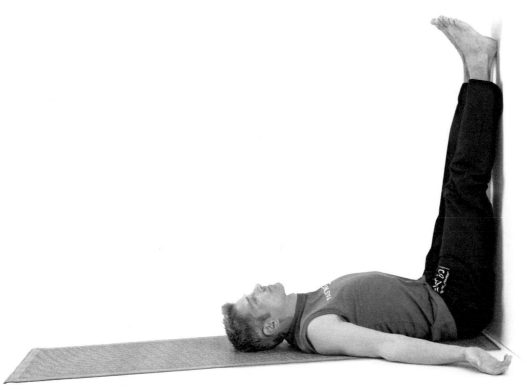

Benefits If your legs are tired from a long day at work or after a long run or workout, you might want to try this easy pose. This is considered a restorative pose in yoga because it restores your body. This pose isn't part of your workout; use it after a hard run or if you were on your feet all day at work.

How do you get into this pose?

- Sit as close to a wall as you can get, with the side of your hip facing the wall.
- Lie down on your side.
- Bring your legs up the wall.

- Bring your palms down by your side.
- Hold for 1 to 3 minutes.

Modify the Pose Bring your hips a little farther from the wall; this will lessen the intensity of the hamstring stretch.

Level of Difficulty This is an easy pose; I would rate it a 5.

QUICK-FIX TIP **Use a blanket under your hips.**

"Yoga for Your Legs" Workout Routine: 10 Minutes

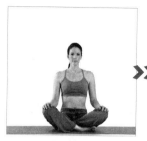

BREATH WORK

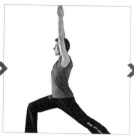

WARRIOR 1 POSE

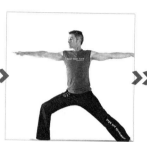

WARRIOR 2 POSE

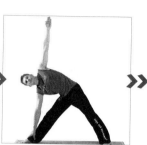

TRIANGLE POSE

Come down to the floor, on your mat if you have one. Sit up tall in an easy cross-legged position and close your eyes. We are going to take a minute to center your body and get you focused on your legs. Take a deep breath in through your nose and exhale it through your mouth. We're going to do this two more times; each time try to hold your breath for a few moments before you exhale.

For the legs workout, we are going to "link poses." If you take a yoga class, you might find yourself doing a series of poses on one side, then doing the same set of poses on the other side. So come to a standing position and bring your legs about 3 to 4 feet apart; depending on your height it may be a shorter or farther distance. Turn your right foot out and turn your left foot slightly in. Bend your knee to a 90-degree angle. Your hips should be squared; try to get them as even as you can. Once you have your legs set, bring your arms to the ceiling with your palms facing each other. This seems like an easy pose until you start to hold it for a while. Make sure your knee is in line with your ankle. Hold for 45 seconds to 1 minute.

From Warrior 1, keep your legs right where they are. Shift your hips so that you are turned to the right. Bring your arms straight out at shoulder level—I want you to feel like you are reaching to the front and the back of the room. Now check your knee; if your hips are tight, your knee may have buckled in. To really work on your legs, keep them active. In this pose, you get the added benefit of working on the flexibility of your hips. Warrior poses are meant to be "strong" poses, and the longer you hold them the harder they become. Hold for 45 seconds to 1 minute.

From Warrior 2, straighten your front leg and reach out with your right hand, then bring your right hand to your shin. If you are more flexible, you can bring your hand to your ankle or to the floor, then bring your left arm to the ceiling. Keep your back foot grounded; don't let the heel come up. Now look up toward your top hand and breathe! Hold for 45 seconds to 1 minute.

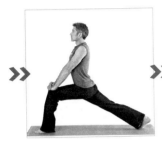

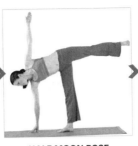

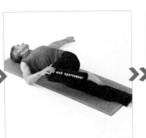

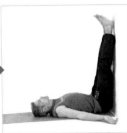

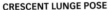

CRESCENT LUNGE POSE

HALF MOON POSE

EASY SPINAL TWIST

LEGS UP A WALL POSE

From Triangle pose, step back to your Warrior 2 pose. This takes core strength, but don't worry, with time you'll get this move. Once you are in Warrior 2 pose, shift your weight onto the ball of your back foot, square off your hips, and bring your hands to your hips. I'm sure by now your legs are getting tired, so just hold this pose for 45 seconds and release it by stepping your left leg to your right and shaking it out. Glad that's over? Wrong! Now you have to switch sides. Repeat the whole thing on the left leg.

Okay, now it's going to get a little more challenging. Bend your front knee, shift your weight forward, and bring your right hand to the floor and your left arm to the ceiling. This is a "balancing" pose, so remember to breathe. Hold for 45 seconds to 1 minute.

Come down to the floor on your back and then hug your knees into your chest. Bring your left knee into your chest and keep your right leg straight on the floor. Bring your left knee across your body while keeping your shoulder blades on the mat (or floor). Look over your left shoulder to complete this twist. Hold for 20 to 30 seconds, then hug both knees into your chest. Switch sides. The right knee comes into your chest, and the left leg goes straight. Bring the right knee across your body and look over your right shoulder to complete the twist on the right side. Take a second to notice the difference from one side to the other. Hold for 20 to 30 seconds, then bring both knees into your chest.

Lie down on your back. Because this is "Yoga for Your Legs," for this version of Corpse pose I want you to put your legs up the wall instead of straight out on the floor. This is a restorative pose for your legs. Bring your arms out by your sides. Close your eyes. Take a deep breath in and exhale. Let your whole body relax, and make sure you focus on your legs. Notice whether there is any tightness in your body, then relax that area. I want you to take a deep breath in, and exhale all the breath out. Do this two more times, focusing on relaxing your body. Stay here for about 2 minutes to get the maximum benefits. After you are completely relaxed, take a deep breath in through your nose and just "sigh" it out. Bend your knees, roll onto your right side for a few seconds, then push yourself up to a comfortable, easy, cross-legged position. Take a second to appreciate the fact that you did something good for yourself today. Your legs will feel refreshed and ready to "run off."

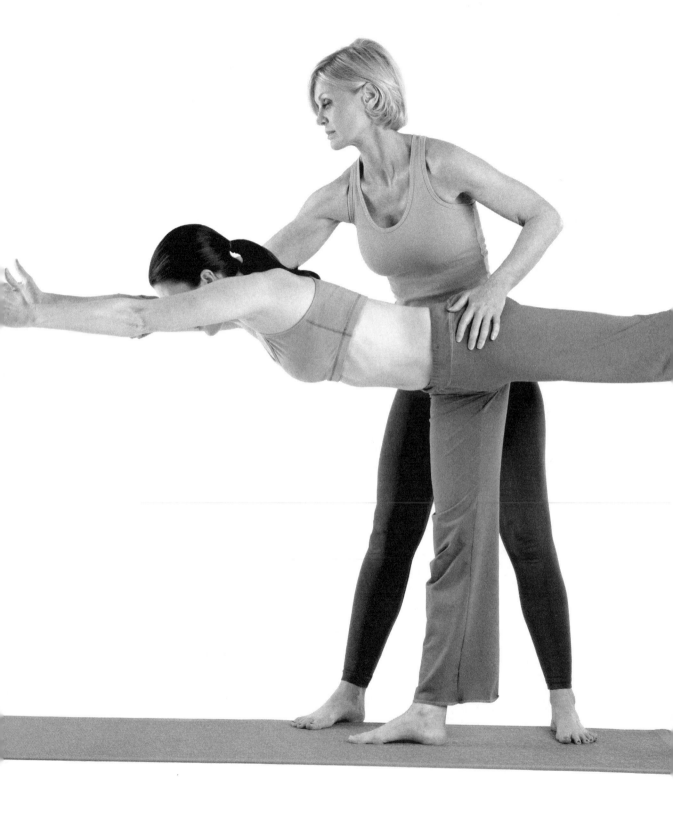

chapter 12

Knees

Weak in the Knees

Your knees are actually hard-working shock absorbers. If you are a runner or play any sports where you have to run, then you definitely know this! Yoga helps keep your knees healthy by lengthening and strengthening the muscles that surround the joints and support your weight. The poses in this section also help mobilize your knee joints by correcting the misalignment that occurs if your muscles are too tight; strength and alignment are the key to healthy knees. Balancing poses are great for the knees because they work on each leg individually; normally the body will compensate for any imbalances in the body, making them worse, not better.

Unfortunately, balancing poses are not the easiest ones to do if you are a beginner, so don't get frustrated if you cannot do them perfectly the first time or two, or maybe three.

I will give you some modifications, easier versions of the poses, that you can use if you are having problems. Don't worry—your balance will improve the longer you practice. Practice makes perfect! (Perfect in this situation would be not to fall over.) In the beginning or on days where you feel "off balance" (and we all have those days), just use a wall for support. Either lean up against a wall or bring your hands to the wall or a chair for support. Remember to breathe! Breath is extremely important in all balancing poses. Breath = balance. I think a good thing to remember in every stressful situation is that when you breathe, you relax.

You may be reading this chapter because you are recovering from a knee injury, or because you know how important your knees are and want to make sure they don't get injured. I'm hoping it's the latter, but I will cover both strengthening your knees and rehabbing them. If you have recently had a knee injury, talk to your doctor before you start the "Yoga for Your Knees" workout routine. This routine can be used to restore flexibility and strengthen the muscles around the knee. Remember, "No pain, no gain" does not apply to yoga, especially when it comes to your knees! So if any of the poses hurt, just don't do them—this goes for when you are using this book, taking a yoga class, or watching a DVD. If you have had an injury to your knee and it is still swelling, wait until the swelling goes away before you start this or any other exercise routine.

In my classes are numerous students who have had issues with their knees. My studio attracts a lot of athletes, and most athletes from a variety of sports deal with knee issues. I have runners, cyclists, soccer players, tennis players, rugby players—you name it, we have it. It's great to get testimonials from students saying that yoga has helped them with their knees, relieving pain and building the muscle around the knees so they can continue to play their sport and stay in the game. That always makes me happy.

So how to protect your knees while doing yoga? Try not to hyperextend your knees; if you already know that you hyperextend your knees, you might want to keep a slight bend in your knees when you are doing standing poses. Watch your form in all your Warrior poses and Side-Angle pose, and don't let the knee buckle in. With these poses, keep the knee in line with your ankle.

For all of you "weekend warriors," the "Yoga for Your Knees" workout is a great routine to use as preventive medicine. Injury prevention is the number one reason athletes do yoga. I get e-mails from people all over the world telling me how my *Yoga for Athletes*® DVD has helped them stay injury-free during their training. Carla from the United Kingdom said that by doing yoga just two times a week, for the first time she didn't hurt herself while training for the London Marathon. When I do my "Yoga for Runners" workshops, I incorporate these poses along with poses from the "Yoga for Your Hips" routine, with some amazing results from the participants: "Best race time ever." "Fastest recovery." "Did not get injured this year."

How Do the Knees Work?

The knee joint may look simple, but it is one of the most complex parts of your body (besides your feet). Unfortunately, the knees are more likely to get injured than any other part of your body, maybe because we rarely pay attention to them until something happens. The knee joint is the largest joint in the body. Understanding a little about the anatomy of the knee joint will help you understand how yoga can help strengthen your knees and keep them from getting injured, especially because knee injuries are the most common sports injury.

Bones of the knee joint: The knee is made up of four main bones: the femur (thighbone), the tibia (shinbone), the fibula (outer shinbone), and the patella (kneecap). The main movements of the knee joint occur between the femur, patella, and tibia. Each of the bones is covered in articular cartilage, an extremely hard, smooth substance designed to decrease the frictional forces as movement occurs between the bones. The patella lies in an indentation at the lower end of the femur known as the intercondylar groove. At the outer surface of the tibia lies the fibula, a long, thin bone that travels right down to the ankle joint.

Ligaments of the knee joint: The knee is stabilized by the ligaments that surround it; each ligament has a different function.

The *medial collateral ligament (MCL)* runs between the inner surfaces of the femur and the tibia. It resists forces acting from the outer surface of the knee.

The *lateral collateral ligament (LCL)* travels from the outer surface of the femur to the head of the fibula. It resists impacts from the inner surface of the knee.

The *anterior cruciate ligament (ACL)* is one of the most important ligaments in the

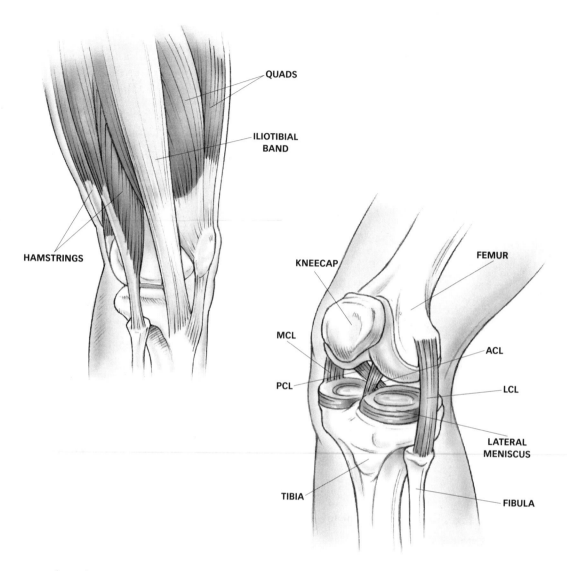

knee because it forms a cross in the middle of the knee joint. The ACL travels from the anterior (front) of the tibia to the posterior (back) of the femur and prevents the tibia from moving forward. It is most commonly injured in twisting movements.

The *posterior cruciate ligament (PCL)* travels from the posterior surface of the tibia to the anterior surface of the femur and in doing so wraps around the ACL.

Menisci (aka knee cartilage): Each knee joint has two crescent-shaped cartilage menisci. These lie on the medial (inner) and lateral (outer) edges of the upper surface of the tibia bone. They act as shock absorbers for the knee, as well as allowing for correct weight distribution between the tibia and the femur.

Iliotibial band: The iliotibial band (ITB) is actually a long tendon. (Tendons connect muscles to bone.) It attaches to a short muscle at the top of the pelvis called the tensor fascia lata. The iliotibial band runs down the side of the thigh and connects to the outside edge of the tibia (shinbone) just below the middle of the knee joint. You can feel the tendon on the outside of your thigh when you tighten your leg muscles. The iliotibial band crosses over the side of the knee joint, giving added stability to the knee.

The lower end of the iliotibial band passes over the outer edge of the lateral femoral condyle, the area where the lower part of the femur (thighbone) bulges out above the knee joint. When the knee is bent and straightened, the tendon glides across the edge of the femoral condyle.

A bursa rests between the femoral condyle and the ITB. Normally, this bursa lets the tendon glide smoothly back and forth over the edge of the femoral condyle as the knee bends and straightens.

Muscle groups surrounding the knee joint: The two main muscle groups of the knee joint are the quadriceps and the hamstrings. The quadriceps consist of four different individual muscles that join to form the quadriceps tendon. This thick tendon connects the muscle to the patella, which in turn connects to the tibia via the patellar tendon. Contraction of the quadriceps pulls the patella upward and leads to knee extension. The hamstrings flex the knee joint and provide stability.

Common Injuries of the Knees

Injuries of the medial and lateral collateral ligaments: These ligaments can be stretched or torn when the foot is planted and a sideways force is directed to the knee. This can cause significant pain and make walking difficult as the body tries to protect the knee, but there is usually little swelling within the knee. The treatment for this injury may include a knee immobilizer, a removable splint that keeps the knee straight and stable.

Injuries of the meniscus: The cartilage of the knee can be acutely injured or can gradually tear. Acutely, the injury is of a twisting nature where the cartilage that is attached to and lays flat on the tibia is pinched between the femoral condyle and the tibial plateau.

Pain and swelling occur gradually over many hours (as opposed to an ACL tear, which swells much more quickly).

The medial meniscus can be torn by twisting the knee violently or by the normal aging process. In either case, the injury causes pain and swelling in the knee and inability to straighten the leg. The two menisci are easily injured by the force of rotating the knee while bearing weight. A partial or total tear of a meniscus may occur when a person quickly twists or rotates the upper leg while the foot stays still (for example, when dribbling a basketball around an opponent or turning to hit a tennis ball). If the tear is tiny, the meniscus stays connected to the front and back of the knee; if the tear is large, the meniscus may be left hanging by a thread of cartilage. The seriousness of a tear depends on its location and extent. Treatment typically involves surgery. The torn portion of the cartilage is removed and the remaining areas are smoothed out during a procedure called a meniscectomy.

ACL injuries: If the foot is planted and force is applied from the front to the back of the knee, the cruciate ligaments can be damaged. The knee swells within minutes, and attempts at walking are difficult. Definitive diagnosis is difficult to establish in the emergency department because the swelling and pain make it hard to test whether the ligament is loose. Long-term treatment may require surgery and significant physical therapy to return good function of the knee joint.

Fractures: Knee bone fractures are relatively common. The patella may fracture from a fall directly onto it or in car accidents in which the knee is driven into the dashboard. The head of the fibula on the lateral side of the knee joint can be fractured by a direct blow or as part of an injury to the shin or ankle. This bone usually heals with little intervention.

Bursa inflammation: Housemaid's knee (prepatellar bursitis) is due to repetitive kneeling and crawling on the knees. A bursa is a fluid-filled sac that cushions body tissues from friction. These sacs are present where muscles or tendons glide against one another. The bursa between the skin and kneecap becomes inflamed and fills with fluid. It is a localized injury and does not involve the knee itself.

Patellar injuries: The kneecap sits within the tendon of the quadriceps muscle, in front of the femur, just above the knee joint. It is held in place by the muscles of the knee. The patella can dislocate laterally toward the outside of the knee. This occurs more commonly in women because of anatomic differences in the angle aligning the femur and tibia. Fortunately, the dislocation is easily returned to the normal position by straightening out the knee, usually resulting in the kneecap popping into place. Patellofemoral syndrome occurs when the underside of the patella becomes inflamed if it does not track smoothly as it rides its path with each flexion and extension of the knee. I see this in a lot of cyclists who come to class. This inflammation can cause localized pain, especially with walking down stairs. Treatment includes ice, anti-inflammatory medication, and exercises to balance the quadriceps muscle (which is what we do in the "Yoga for Your Knees" workout).

Iliotibial band syndrome: The iliotibial band glides back and forth over the lateral femoral condyle as the knee bends and straightens. Normally, this isn't a problem. The bursa between the lateral femoral condyle and the ITB can become irritated and inflamed if the ITB starts to snap over the condyle with repeated knee motions, such as those from walking, running, or biking.

People often end up with iliotibial band syndrome from overdoing their activity or sport. This overuse problem is often seen in cyclists, runners, and long-distance walkers. It causes pain on the outside of the knee, just above the joint. It rarely gets so bad that it requires surgery, but it can be "a pain." They try to push themselves too far, too fast, and they end up running, walking, or biking more than their body can handle. The repeated strain causes the bursa on the side of the knee to become inflamed.

Some experts believe that the problem happens when the knee bows outward. This can happen in runners if their shoes are worn on the outside edge, or if they run on slanted terrain. Others feel that certain foot abnormalities, such as foot pronation, cause iliotibial band syndrome. (Pronation of the foot occurs when the arch flattens.)

Runners with a weakened or fatigued gluteus medius muscle in the hip are more likely to end up with iliotibial band syndrome. This muscle controls outward movements of the hip. If the gluteus medius isn't doing its job, the thigh tends to turn inward. This makes the knee angle into a knock-kneed position. The iliotibial band becomes tightened against the bursa on the side of the knee.

What does iliotibial band syndrome feel like? The symptoms of the syndrome commonly begin with pain over the outside of the knee, just above the knee joint. Tenderness in this area is usually worse after activity. As the bursitis grows worse, pain may radiate up the side of the thigh and down the side of the leg. My students sometimes tell me they hear a snapping or popping sensation on the outside of the knee.

Arthritis: The best way to prevent and treat arthritis in your knees is to "keep moving." When we start to have joint pain, we often stop moving, which starts this vicious circle. We should apply the "move it or lose it" motto to arthritis. Most doctors recommend an exercise routine that promotes flexibility and strengthening to decrease the pain of arthritis. Yoga is the perfect remedy because it both helps with flexibility and strength but also provides a no-impact workout. Rheumatoid arthritis is actually aggravated by stress; because yoga is a great stress reliever, it can help reduce the pain of rheumatoid arthritis and promote healing of the joints.

The following yoga poses help your knees stay strong and flexible. As you can see from "How Do the Knees Work?" they are affected by the muscles in your legs and hips; when you are doing the "Yoga for Your Legs" or "Yoga for Your Hips" workouts, you are also helping your knees.

POSES TO HELP YOUR KNEES:

1. Chair pose

2. Tree pose

3. Warrior 3 pose

4. Hero's pose

Chair Pose

QUICK-FIX TIP

Pay attention to how far you go down on the wall so you can mark your progress as you do the "Yoga for Your Knees" workout.

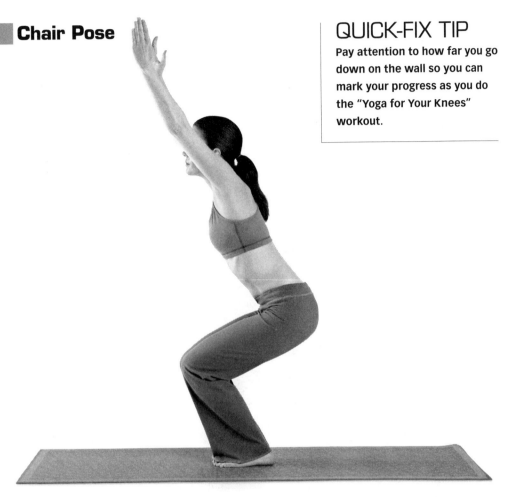

Benefits Chair works on all the muscles that support the knees. The modified version we are going to do will also open the iliotibial band, which affects a lot of runners. Because the iliotibial band runs from your hip to just below the knee, doing this pose will help prevent it from getting inflamed.

How do you get into this pose?

- Begin with your feet together.
- Place your back up against the wall.
- Bring your legs together.

- Squat down, making sure to keep your spine long and your chest open.
- Bring your arms alongside your ears.
- Hold for 45 seconds to 1 minute.

Modify the Pose To make this pose a little easier, bring your legs about hip-distance apart; don't go down as far.

Level of Difficulty Chair pose can be a hard pose. I would give it a 7.

Tree Pose

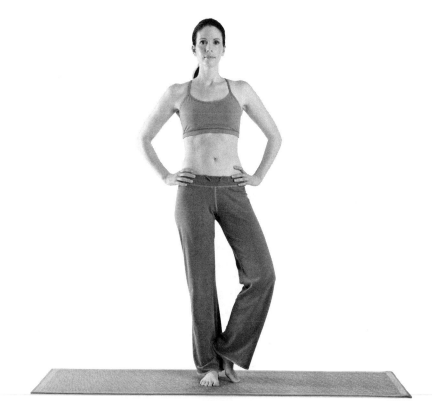

Benefits Tree pose is a classic yoga pose, one I'm sure you have heard of—or at least you might recognize the picture. It is one of the easier balancing poses; that's why we are going to start with it. Then we'll move on to the harder balancing poses. Tree pose strengthens the muscles around your knees.

How do you get into this pose?

- Come to a standing position.
- Put your hands on your hips and balance on your right foot.
- Bring your left foot to the inside of your right thigh. You can grab your ankle with your hand and place it to the inside of your thigh.
- Press your foot into your thigh to move the bent knee out to the side.
- Try to keep your hips even.
- Bring your hands together in what is called prayer position, in front of your chest.
- Find a focus point.
- Hold for 45 seconds to 1 minute.
- Switch sides.
- Balance on your left foot.
- Bring your right foot to the inside of your thigh.
- Place your hands in prayer position at your chest.

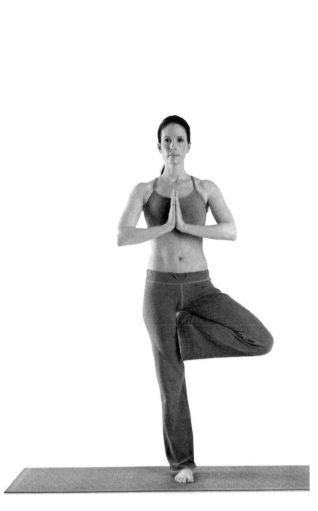

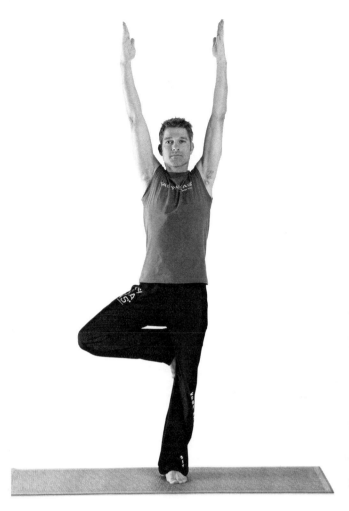

- If you feel secure in that position and want to challenge yourself, lift your arms above your head.
- Hold for 45 seconds to 1 minute.

Modify the Pose If this pose is too challenging right now, drop the raised foot to the calf or put the big toe on the ground. You can also bring your hand to the wall for support. Try not to hyperextend your knees. It's also good to use a wall for support if your knees aren't that strong or you are rehabbing from an injury.

Level of Difficulty This is one of the easier balancing poses, but it's still a balancing pose—I rate it a 7.

QUICK-FIX TIP Sometimes students have a hard time keeping the foot of the bent leg to the inside of the thigh; make sure you are wearing something that's not slippery, like cotton sweats, so your foot will have some traction on the fabric. If you are wearing shorts, make sure you don't have lotion on your legs—your foot will slip right off.

Warrior 3 Pose

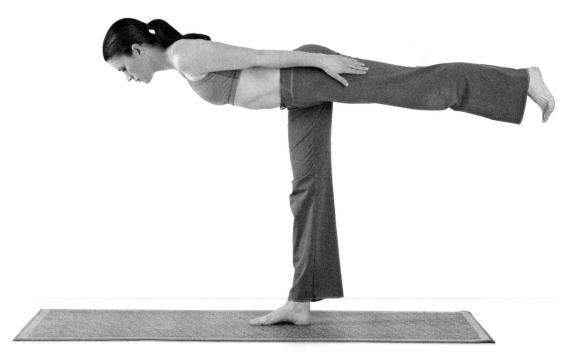

Benefits Warrior 3 helps build strength in your legs while improving your balance and concentration. This is not an easy pose.

How do you get into this pose?

- Stand up.
- Balance on your right leg.
- Hinge forward at your hips.
- Bring your left leg up to hip level.
- Keep the knee of your raised leg facing the floor.

- Bring your arms out in front of you. If this is too difficult, keep them by your sides, as shown above.
- Bring your body into a T formation.
- Keep your hips square and level to the floor.
- Find a focus point in front of you.
- Hold for 45 seconds to 1 minute.
- Repeat on the left leg.

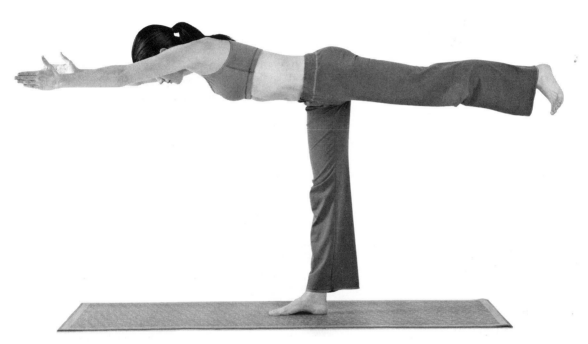

Modify the Pose If this pose is too challenging right now, do it close to a wall. For stability, place both of your hands on the wall for support. You still get all the benefits of the pose. In fact, to strengthen the knee, you can really focus on the leg you are standing on, and you may be able to hold this pose longer. I give this option to a lot of the athletes I train, so don't feel like you are wimping out by modifying this pose.

Level of Difficulty This is one of the harder balancing poses; I would definitely give it at least an 8.5.

QUICK-FIX TIP Sometimes
having a focus point helps with balance, especially if you are a visual person. My Venice, California, studio has brick walls, and I encourage my students to "pick a brick" during balancing postures. Remember, it's okay to fall, as long as you get back up and try it again!

Hero's Pose

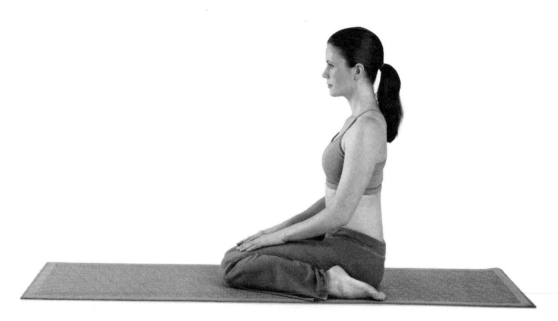

Benefits Hero's pose stretches the muscles around the knees. There are a lot of schools of thought in the yoga community about Hero's pose, but most find this pose beneficial. I personally find it very helpful for your knees and use it in my *Yoga for Athletes*® video. If you do have a knee injury, ask your doctor first before doing any of these poses.

How do you get into this pose?

- Drop down to your knees.
- Bring your knees together.

- Bring your feet straight back behind you, a little wider than your hips; your heels should touch the outside of your hips.
- Your toes and the tops of your feet should be flat on the floor.
- Sit back between your feet.
- Bring your chest up, sit up straight.
- Place your hands on your thighs.
- Hold for 45 seconds to 1 minute.

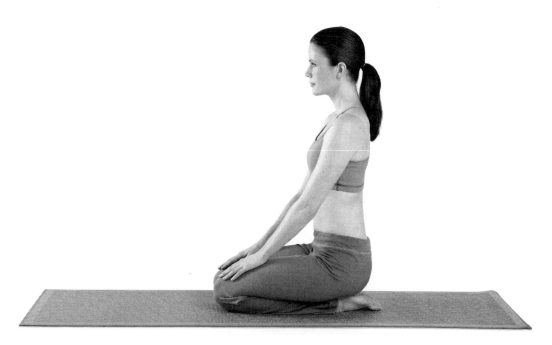

Modify the Pose If your butt does not hit the floor, then you will want to modify this pose. You can sit up on a block if you have one, or use one or two folded blankets.

Level of Difficulty If your knees or the muscles around your knees are tight, this can be a really hard pose. I would rate it a solid 6.

QUICK-FIX TIP **Make sure you are on a rug or a padded surface for Hero's pose. A common mistake I see in class is students bringing their feet out to the sides instead of straight back by their hips, so make sure your toes are pointing straight back to protect your knees.**

"Yoga for Your Knees" Workout Routine: 10 Minutes

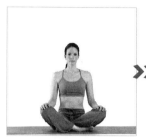 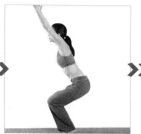 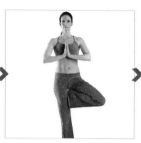 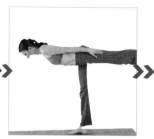

BREATH WORK

CHAIR POSE

TREE POSE

WARRIOR 3 POSE

Sit in an easy cross-legged position, sit up tall, and close your eyes. We are going to take a minute to center your body and get you focused on your knees. Take a deep breath in through your nose and exhale it through your mouth. We're going to do this two more times; each time, try to hold your breath for a few moments before you exhale.

For this Chair pose, we are going to use a wall for support. Find a wall that you can lean up against. Bring your back up against the wall, then start to lower your hips until they are knee level. It's like you are sitting on an invisible chair. Your feet should be together; if that's too hard, bring your feet about hip-distance apart. Bring your hands to your thighs. Hold for 45 seconds to 1 minute. You will probably feel a little burn in your thigh muscles. This is a great pose for those of you who ski.

Come to a standing position. Balance on your right foot. Bring your left foot to the inside of your right thigh. You can grab your ankle with your hand and place it to the inside of your thigh. Press your foot into your thigh to move the bent knee out to the side. Try to keep your hips even. Bring your hands together in what is called prayer position, in front of your chest. Find a focus point. Hold for 45 seconds to 1 minute. Switch sides, and balance on your left foot. Bring your right foot to the inside of your thigh. Place your hands in prayer position at your chest. Hold for 45 seconds to 1 minute.

Stay standing. Balance on your right leg. Hinge forward at your hips. Bring your left leg up to hip level. Keep the knee of your raised leg facing the floor. Bring your arms out in front of you. Bring your body into a T formation. Keep your hips square and level to the floor. Find a focus point in front of you. Hold for 45 seconds to 1 minute. Repeat on the left leg.

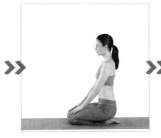

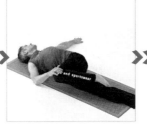

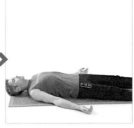

HERO'S POSE

EASY SPINAL TWIST

CORPSE POSE

Drop down to your knees and bring your knees together. Bring your feet straight back behind you, a little wider than your hips; your heels should touch the outside of your hips. Your toes and the tops of your feet should be flat on the floor. Sit back between your feet. Bring your chest up and sit up straight. Place your hands on your thighs. Hold for 45 seconds to 1 minute. If you find that your butt is not hitting the floor, then sit up on your feet.

From Hero's pose, just shift your weight onto your side and roll down onto your back, then hug your knees into your chest. Bring your left knee into your chest and straighten your right leg on the floor. Bring your left knee across your body while keeping your shoulder blades on the mat (or floor). Look over your left shoulder to complete this twist. Hold for 20 to 30 seconds, then hug both knees into your chest. Switch sides. The right knee comes into your chest, and the left leg goes straight. Bring the right knee across your body and look over your right shoulder to complete the twist on the right side. Take a second to notice the difference from one side to the other. Hold for 20 to 30 seconds, then bring both knees into your chest.

Take a deep breath in; on your exhale, just let your whole body come to the floor. Bring your arms out by your sides with your palms up. Remember, don't skip this part; it helps the body adjust to what you just did. It allows the benefits of your workout to sink in before you run off. Close your eyes and try to let your whole body relax. Notice whether there is any tightness in your body, and relax that area. Take a deep breath in, pretend that you are breathing from your feet, and bring the breath all the way through your body and exhale it all out. Repeat two more times. Stay here for about 2 minutes to get the maximum benefits. Take a deep breath in through your nose and just "sigh" it out. Bend your knees, roll onto your right side for a few seconds, and push yourself up to a comfortable, easy, cross-legged position. Bring your hands together in front of your chest, take a deep breath in, and on your exhale bow forward. Take a second to appreciate the fact that you did something good for yourself today. Your knees will thank you!

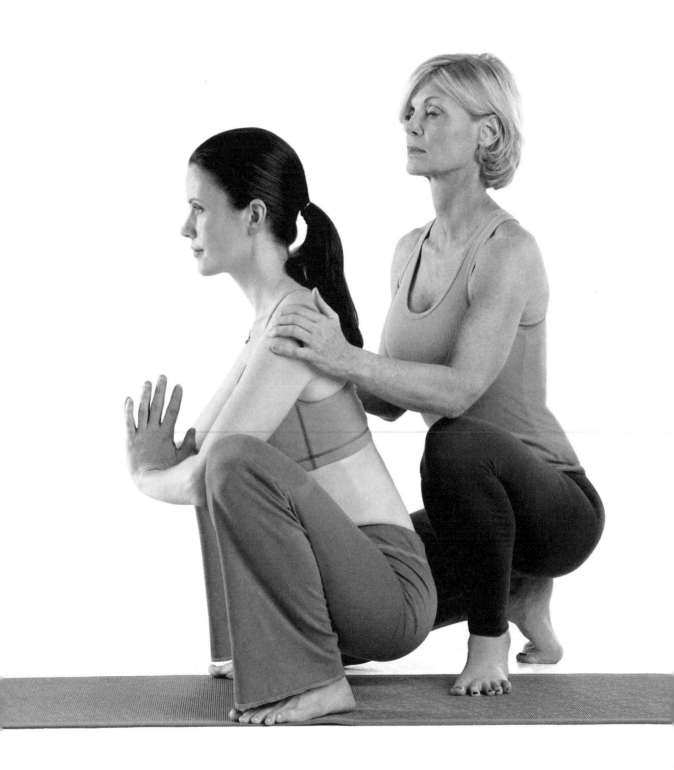

chapter 13

Feet and Ankles

Treat Your Feet

I have to admit, I find feet one of the most fascinating parts of the body. They have more bones—26, in fact—than any other part of your body. Without them you don't walk, run, or do just about any sport. Think about it: When your feet hurt, it affects your whole body, right? For yoga, you use your feet in just about every standing pose—"the flow" section of a class. Poses such as Mountain, Standing Forward Bend, and Warrior, just to name a few, work on strengthening your feet and ankles. Correct alignment of the feet in all yoga poses is important. I can definitely attest to the fact that yoga helps strengthen the feet. After years of practicing yoga, my feet are strong and my balance is great. My toes spread wide in Warrior 3, which is great for balance but not the best look in sandals!

It doesn't matter whether you are walking the streets of New York City or running along the coast of California, your feet are taking a pounding. We won't talk about wearing heels—I can tell instantly the students in my class who wear heels because their toes are pointed and there isn't any flexion in their feet. Guys don't have this issue (well, most guys). Eighty percent of all foot problems are in women, mostly because of their shoes. I am not saying don't wear heels; instead, just do some yoga.

Now, yoga is a barefoot practice, no matter how many athletic shoe companies try to get you to wear "yoga shoes"—crazy, isn't it? Being barefoot also counterbalances the pressure and strain you put on your feet by wearing tight shoes. When you practice yoga, you use all the muscles in your feet; it not only strengthens them but also helps maintain healthy arches. Maybe this is because I teach yoga and see feet all day, but I love seeing "pretty" feet. I actually go into the care of your feet in my teachers' training; there is nothing worse than a yoga instructor with bad feet. You can tell people who care about themselves because they care about their feet. If you want to "give your feet a treat," try reflexology, a massage that encourages overall health by stimulating other parts of your body.

If you think about it, everything starts with your feet; they are the first thing that hits the floor when you get out of bed. If your feet hurt or are tired, your body feels tired. A lot of health issues first become visible by showing signs in your feet, like diabetes, arthritis, and circulatory conditions, just to name a few. So pay more attention to your feet. Our feet are our foundation; the body lines up over the feet. If your foot goes out of alignment, so will the ankle, hips, and back. Lots of lower back and hip pain starts with the feet.

For those of you who are runners, think about how much running books focus on your feet, foot strike, and how the foot rolls when you run. It's all about the alignment of your feet and the distribution of your weight when you run—this also affects your ankles, knees, hips, back, and shoulders.

How Do the Feet Work?

Each foot has 26 bones, 33 muscles, 31 joints, and over 100 ligaments. In fact, the feet contain 25% of all the bones in the body. I don't know about you, but I find that fascinating. Another fascinating, but slightly disturbing, fact is that the feet contain 250,000 sweat glands—so you can see why your feet sweat!

Our poor feet are constantly under stress. It's no wonder that 80% of us will have some sort of problem with our feet at some time or another. Many things affect the condition of our feet: activity level, occupation, other health conditions, and, most important, shoes (especially shoes with high heels). Many of the problems that arise in the foot are directly related to shoes, so it is very important to choose shoes that are good for your feet; this means wearing the right size—if you are an 8½, why buy a size 8 shoe?

The foot is an incredibly complex mechanism. I'm not going to go into it in detail, just enough to help you understand how important feet are and how yoga can help them. The

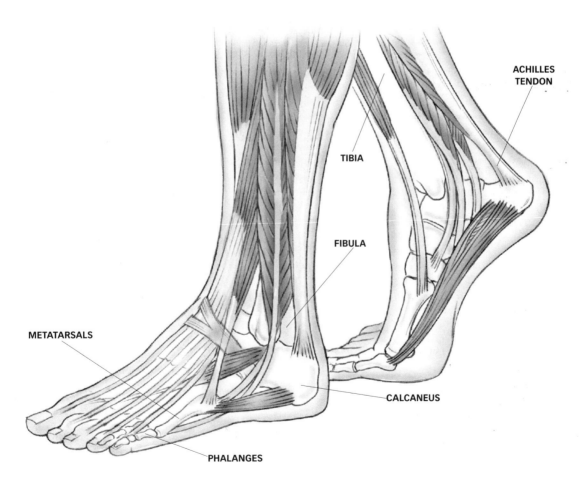

important structures and functions of the feet can be divided into several categories, which include the bones and joints, ligaments and tendons, muscles, nerves, and blood vessels. Let's take a quick look at each of them.

Bones and joints: The skeleton of the foot begins with the talus, which is your ankle-bone. The two bones of the lower leg, the large tibia and the smaller fibula, come together at the ankle to form a very stable structure known as a mortise-and-tenon joint. The two bones that make up the back part of the foot are the talus and the calcaneus, the heel bone. The talus is connected to the calcaneus at the subtalar joint. The ankle joint allows the foot to bend up and down. The subtalar joint allows the foot to rock from side to side.

Just down the foot from the ankle is a set of five bones called tarsal bones, which work together as a group. These bones are unique in the way they fit together. There are multiple joints between the tarsal bones. When the foot is twisted in one direction by the muscles of the foot and leg, these bones lock together and form a very rigid structure. When they are twisted in the opposite direction, they become unlocked and allow the foot to conform to whatever surface the foot is contacting, whether sidewalk or beach sand. The tarsal bones are connected to the five long bones of the foot, called the metatarsals.

Finally, there are the bones of the toes, the phalanges. The joints between the metatarsals and the first phalanx is called the metatarsophalangeal joint (MTP). These joints form the ball of the foot, and movement in these joints is very important for walking. Not much motion occurs at the joints between the bones of the toes. The big toe, the hallux, is the most important toe for walking, and the first MTP joint is a common area for problems in the foot.

Ligaments and tendons: Ligaments are the soft tissues that attach bone to bone. Ligaments are very similar to tendons. The difference is that tendons attach muscles to bones. Both of these structures consist of small fibers of a material called collagen. The collagen fibers are bundled together to form a rope-like structure. Ligaments and tendons come in many different sizes, and like rope, are made up of many smaller fibers. The thicker the ligament or tendon, the stronger it is.

The large Achilles tendon is the most important tendon for walking, running, and jumping. It attaches the calf muscles to the heel bone to allow us to raise up on our toes. The posterior tibial tendon attaches one of the smaller muscles of the calf to the underside of the foot. This tendon helps support the arch and allows us to turn the foot inward. The toes have tendons attached that bend the toes down (on the bottom of the toes) and straighten the toes (on the top of the toes). The anterior tibial tendon allows us to raise the foot. Two tendons run behind the outer bump of the ankle, which is called the lateral malleolus, and help turn the foot outward.

Many small ligaments hold the bones of the foot together. Most of these ligaments form part of the joint capsule around each joint of the foot. A joint capsule is a watertight sac that forms around all joints. It is made up of the ligaments around the joint and the soft tissues between the ligaments that fill in the gaps and form the sac.

Muscles: Most of the motion of the foot is caused by the muscles in the lower leg. Contraction of the leg muscles is the main way that we move our feet. There are numerous small muscles in the foot. While these muscles are not nearly as important as the small muscles in the hand, they do affect the way that the toes work. Most of the muscles of the foot are arranged in layers on the sole of the foot, which is called the plantar surface. There they connect to and move the toes, as well as provide padding underneath the sole of the foot.

Nerves: The main nerve to the foot, the tibial nerve, enters the sole of the foot by running behind the inside bump on the ankle, the medial malleolus. This nerve supplies sensation to the toes and sole of the foot. Several other nerves run on the outside of the foot and down the top of the foot. These nerves primarily provide sensation to different areas on the top and outside edges of the foot.

Blood vessels: The main blood supply to the foot, the posterior tibial artery, runs right beside the nerve of the same name. Other less important arteries enter the foot from other directions. One of these arteries is the dorsalis pedis, which runs down the top of the foot. You can feel your pulse where this artery runs down the top of the foot.

As you can see, the anatomy and function of the foot is very complex. When everything works together, the foot functions correctly. But when one part becomes damaged, it can affect every other part of the foot and lead to problems. You can see why we really need to take care of our feet!

Common Foot and Ankle Injuries

Achilles tendinitis: This condition is inflammation of the Achilles tendon, which extends down the back of the leg from the calf muscles to the heel. It can become inflamed from overuse and inflexibility. An inflamed Achilles tendon feels tender and stiff. Running tends to tighten the calf muscle. When the muscle becomes too tight, it doesn't allow for the normal biomechanics of running, and the Achilles tendon becomes strained and inflamed. Running steep hills or increasing your weekly mileage too quickly can lead to inflammation of the tendon. If you continue to run despite the pain, the inflammation can turn into partial tears of the tendon. Eventually, part of the tendon will die, and the weakened remaining tendon can easily rupture.

Ankle sprains: Sprains result in pain and swelling and occur when some of the ligaments surrounding the ankle (usually on the outside of the joint) are torn or stretched. As these tears heal, they form scar tissue, which sticks to normal tissue and causes inflammation and continued pain. Without appropriate treatment, ankle pain can persist for months, even years. Runners most commonly sprain ankles by stepping in a pothole or tripping on a tree root, but balancing poses will help you prevent this.

Blisters: Blisters are the accumulation of fluid between the skin's inner and outer layers. They are rarely serious, but if not treated they can become infected and force a layoff from running. Prolonged friction between your foot, socks, and shoes creates blisters. I always tell my students who are runners to put petroleum jelly on their feet before they run and to wear two pairs of socks. This really does help.

Bunions: A bunion is a bony growth on the side of the base of your big toe. Pressure from your shoe and motion at the joint can cause pain. Bunions gradually become worse until running or even walking becomes extremely painful. A bunion is an arthritic condition that can result from a genetic defect or biomechanical problems, such as overpronation or tight-fitting shoes.

Plantar fasciitis: Plantar fasciitis is one of the most common foot ailments among runners. It usually begins as a tenderness or mild pain on the sole of your foot near the arch or heel. Gradually it becomes more severe and localizes to a spot under your heel that feels like a bone bruise. You'll find that your foot hurts first thing in the morning but feels better as it warms up during the day. The plantar fascia is a ligament-like tissue that runs from the ball of your foot along the arch and inserts into the heel bone. If you have flat feet or if you run with too much foot motion (overpronate), the plantar fascia becomes strained, with most of the stress occurring at the heel.

Stress fractures: Stress fractures are partial breaks or cracks in a bone. In the feet, stress fractures usually occur in the second, third, or fourth metatarsals (toes). It will hurt to touch the top of your foot; if it doesn't, you probably don't have a stress fracture. Stress fractures result from chronic stress to the bone, usually from prolonged overtraining, increasing the load on the bone, adding speedwork, switching from trail running to sidewalks, wearing less supportive shoes, or increasing the number of times the bone is stressed (that is, increasing your mileage). Running causes more stress fractures than any other sport because we tend to run on hard surfaces and land with a force that is four to six times our body weight. Do the math—that's a lot of weight!

POSES TO HELP YOUR FEET AND ANKLES:

1. Mountain pose
2. Eagle pose
3. Standing Forward Bend pose
4. Chair pose
5. Squat pose (aka Garland pose)
6. Reclining Big-Toe pose

Mountain Pose

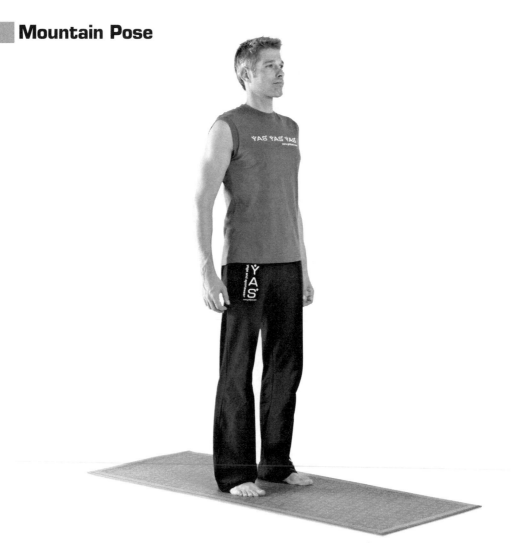

Benefits This pose strengthens the muscles in your feet and helps your balance and posture. It also helps increase muscle tone and stretch of the muscles in your legs. Maintaining good muscle tone in your feet will improve the overall health of your feet and ankles. If you have calluses, it may mean that you have been misusing your feet. Yoga will help, but if you are having serious problems with your feet you should go to a podiatrist.

How do you get into this pose?
- Start in a standing position.
- Bring your feet together.
- Just let your arms hang at your sides, with your palms facing your body.
- Ground your feet into the mat, spread your toes, and concentrate on all four corners of your feet.
- Stand up straight.

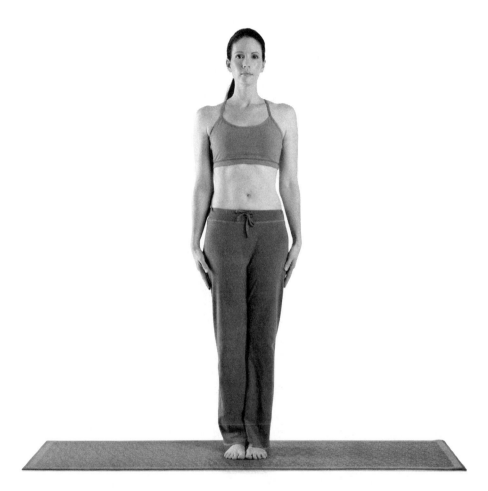

- Stay balanced; don't tilt your hips forward or back.

Modify the Pose Stand up against a wall for support.

Level of Difficulty This is an easy pose for almost everyone; I would rate it a 4.

QUICK-FIX TIP Make sure you are equally distributing your weight between each foot. Take a second to notice whether you favor one foot over the other. When your toes are spread wide, you are activating all the muscles in your feet.

Eagle Pose

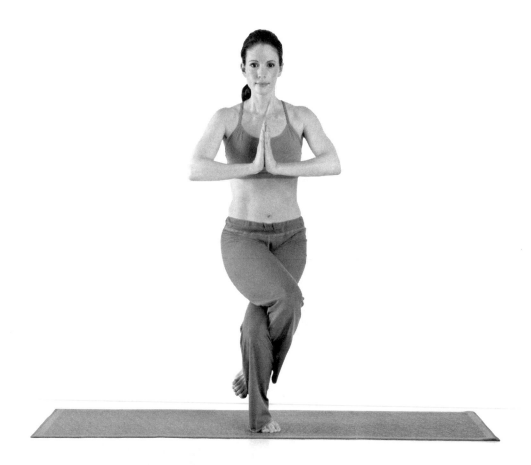

Benefits My students who surf love this pose. They tell me it really helps their balance on their surfboards. This pose is great for a lot of sports, but most people find it challenging. So if you can't do it on your first try, don't worry about it. This pose may be the exception to the "No Pretzel Zone."

How do you get into this pose?

■ Stand on your left leg.

■ Bend your right leg over your left.

■ Bring your right leg up around behind your standing leg.

■ Hook your foot and ankle around behind your calf.

■ Sink down as if you were going to sit on a chair.

■ Move your arms to a prayer position in front of your chest. (You can add the "Eagle arms" to make it more challenging.)

■ Hold for 45 seconds to 1 minute.

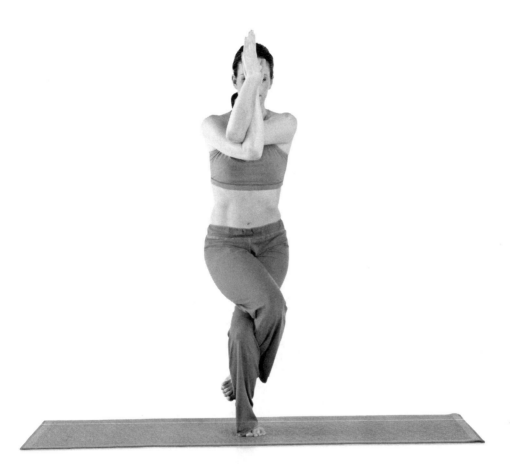

- Come out of the pose and shake out your legs.
- Switch sides.
- To add the "Eagle arms" and come into the full pose, bring your left arm straight out in front of you, bring your right arm under your right, bend your arms at the elbow, and try to bring your palms together in front of your face. (It sounds more complicated than it is.)

Modify the Pose Do the legs only, bringing your hands to the wall for balance.

Level of Difficulty Full Eagle is extremely hard; I rate this pose a 9.

QUICK-FIX TIP Pick a focus point on the wall in front of you. This will help you stay balanced in this pose. The most important thing to do in all the balancing poses is *breathe*.

Standing Forward Bend Pose

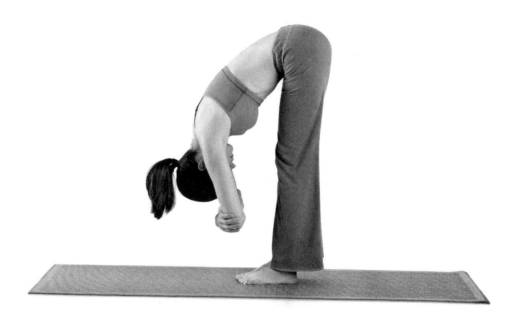

Benefits In the yoga world, Standing Forward Bend is said to have a lot of benefits, from curing depression to relieving the symptoms of menopause. Maybe you're depressed because you are in menopause? But on just a physical level, this pose helps stretch your hamstrings while it strengthens your thighs and knees. Tight hamstrings pull on your lower back, so releasing them also releases your lower back.

How do you get into this pose?

- Stand up straight.
- Bring your legs about hip-distance apart.
- Hinge forward from your hips.
- Clasp opposite elbows.
- Release your neck and let your head hang.
- Hold for 30 seconds to 1 minute.

Modify the Pose You can lean up against the wall.

Level of Difficulty This is an easy pose—I would rate it a 5.

QUICK-FIX TIP Keep your knees bent to release your lower back.

Chair Pose

QUICK-FIX TIP To really get the benefits of Chair pose, keep your weight back into your heels, to the point where your toes pop up. This way you will know that you are also working on your core strength.

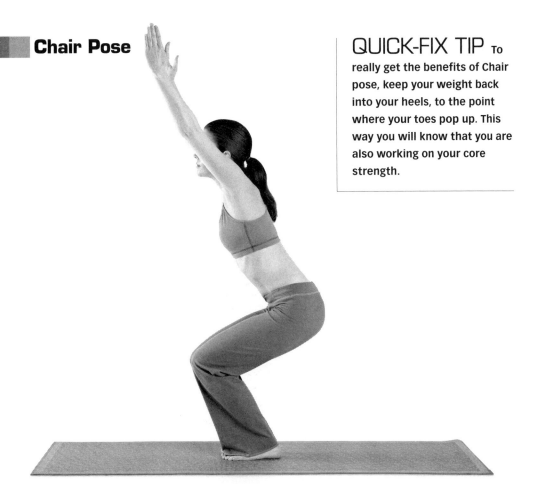

Benefits This pose is supposed to help with "flat feet." It strengthens your feet, ankles, thighs, and calves.

How do you get into this pose?

- Start standing.
- Bring your feet together, legs touching.
- Bring your arms over your head with your palms facing each other.
- Sink your hips back and down; try to get your thighs parallel to the floor.
- Drop your shoulder blades down your back.
- Keep your weight back into your heels to really work on your feet.
- Hold for 30 seconds to 1 minute.

Modify the Pose Do Chair pose up against a wall, as we did in the "Yoga for Your Knees" workout (Chapter 12). If you want to make this pose harder, then stay in Chair pose but come up on your tiptoes for Tiptoe pose. Bring your arms out in front of you and then lower as far as you can go. Hold for 30 seconds to 1 minute.

Level of Difficulty This is not an easy pose, so I would give it at least a 7.5.

Squat Pose (aka Garland Pose)

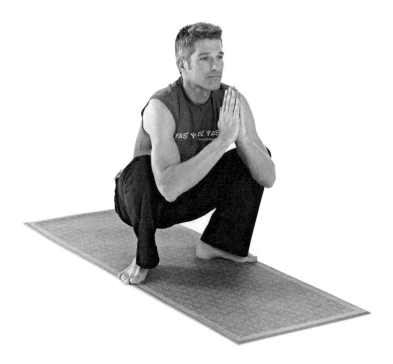

Benefits This pose opens the Achilles tendons to make the feet and ankles more flexible; it also strengthens the arches of the feet and the ankles. If you can get into the pose and your Achilles tendon is flexible, this pose also releases your lower back area and your hips.

How do you get into this pose?

■ Bring your feet about hip-distance apart.

■ Squat down as far as you can.

■ Bring your hands together in front of your chest.

■ Hold for 45 seconds to 1 minute.

Modify the Pose Place a blanket under your heels.

Level of Difficulty Okay, this is one of those poses that is really easy for me. I could sit in this position all day long, but for a lot of you this might be a really hard pose, especially if you have tight Achilles tendons. So I would rate it an 8.

QUICK-FIX TIP **As you lower down into the squat, keep your arms out in front of you for balance.**

Reclining Big-Toe Pose

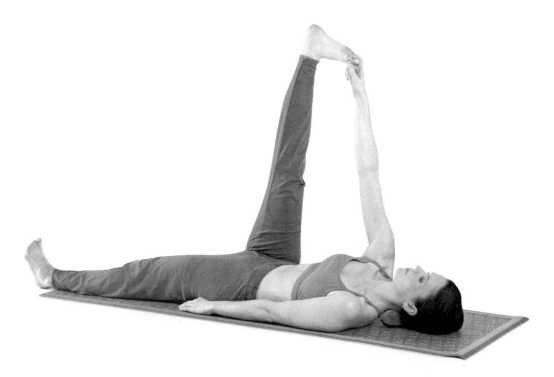

Benefits This pose strengthens the arches of your feet, but it also opens the hamstrings and the psoas in your hip.

How do you get into this pose?

■ Lie down on the floor.

■ Bend the right knee and grab your right toe with your right hand.

■ Keep the left leg on the floor.

■ Make sure your shoulder blades are on the floor.

■ Lift your right leg toward the ceiling.

■ Hold for 45 seconds to 1 minute.

■ Switch sides.

Modify the Pose If you cannot hold on to your toe and keep your leg straight, then use a strap or a towel by wrapping it over your foot.

Level of Difficulty This is a fairly easy pose; I would give it a 5.

QUICK-FIX TIP **Keep your bottom leg pressed into the floor for support.**

"Yoga for Your Feet/Ankles" Workout Routine: 10 Minutes

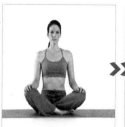

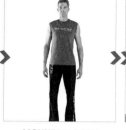

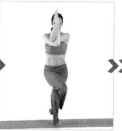

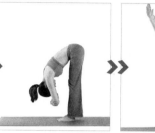

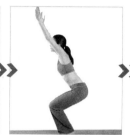

BREATH WORK

MOUNTAIN POSE

EAGLE POSE

STANDING FORWARD BEND POSE

CHAIR POSE

Sit up tall in an easy cross-legged position and close your eyes. We are going to take a minute to center your body and get you focused on your feet and ankles. Take a deep breath in through your nose and exhale through your mouth. Repeat two times.

Start in a standing position with your feet together. Concentrate on all four corners of your feet. Make sure you are distributing your weight evenly between your heels and your toes and between one leg and the other. This pose can tell you a lot about the imbalances in your body, if you pay attention. Don't let your back sway or your hips come forward. If you are having a hard time standing up straight, or if you're not sure if you are, then stand up against a wall. Just let your arms hang by your sides, with your palms facing your body. Remember to breathe. Hold for 1 minute. If you really want to challenge yourself, come up onto your toes.

Now the fun begins. I know I said I would not turn you into a pretzel, but this pose comes close. Stay standing, and balance on your left leg. Bend your right leg over your left. Bring your right leg up and around, behind your standing leg. Hook your foot and ankle around so that they are behind your calf. Sink down as if you were going to sit on a chair. Arms come to prayer position in front of your chest. Hold for 45 seconds to 1 minute. Come out of the pose and shake out your legs. Switch sides. To add the "Eagle arms" and come into the full pose, bring your left arm straight out in front of you, then bring your right arm under your left; bend your arms at the elbow and try to bring your palms together in front of your face.

Bring your feet about hip-distance apart and just hinge forward from your hips. Hold for 45 seconds to 1 minute.

Roll up to standing and bring your legs together, feet touching. Sink your hips down as if you were just about to sit on a chair, then bring your arms to the ceiling, palms facing each other, chest up. Put weight back into your heels—really feel your feet. Come to a standing position.

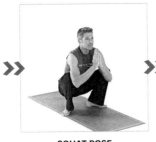 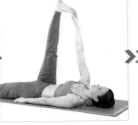 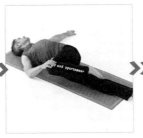 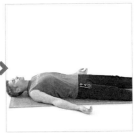

SQUAT POSE

RECLINING BIG-TOE POSE

EASY SPINAL TWIST

CORPSE POSE

Bring your feet about hip-distance apart, sink your hips, and come into a squatting position.

From your Squat pose, just lie down on the floor. Bend the right knee and grab your right toe with your right hand. If you can't reach your foot, then use a strap or a towel. Keep the left leg on the floor. Make sure your shoulder blades are on the floor. Lift your right leg toward the ceiling. Hold for 45 seconds to 1 minute. Really focus on stretching your foot and ankle in this pose. Switch legs.

Hug your knees into your chest. Bring your left knee into your chest and keep your right leg straight on the floor. Bring your left knee across your body while keeping your shoulder blades on the floor. Look over your left shoulder to complete this twist. Hold for 20 to 30 seconds. Hug both knees into your chest and switch sides. The right knee comes into your chest, and the left leg goes straight. Bring the right knee across your body and look over your right shoulder to complete the twist on the right side. Take a second to notice the difference from one side to the other. Hold for 20 to 30 seconds, then bring both knees into your chest.

From here we are going into our final pose, Corpse pose. Stay on your back and bring your arms out by your sides. Close your eyes (if you want, put a towel over your eyes to help you relax). Take a deep breath in through your nose; on your next exhale, let everything go to the floor. We are going to end this workout like we started it, with a little breath work. Remember, don't skip this pose; it helps the body adjust to what you just did. It allows the benefits of your routine to sink into your body before you run off. Let your whole body relax, and make sure you focus on your feet and ankles. I want you to take a deep breath in, and bring the breath all the way through your body and exhale. Repeat two times. Stay here for about 2 minutes. After you are completely relaxed, take a deep breath in through your nose and just "sigh" it out. Bend your knees and roll onto your right side for a few seconds. Push yourself up to a comfortable, easy, cross-legged position. Take a second to appreciate the fact that you did something good for yourself today. Your feet will definitely thank you!

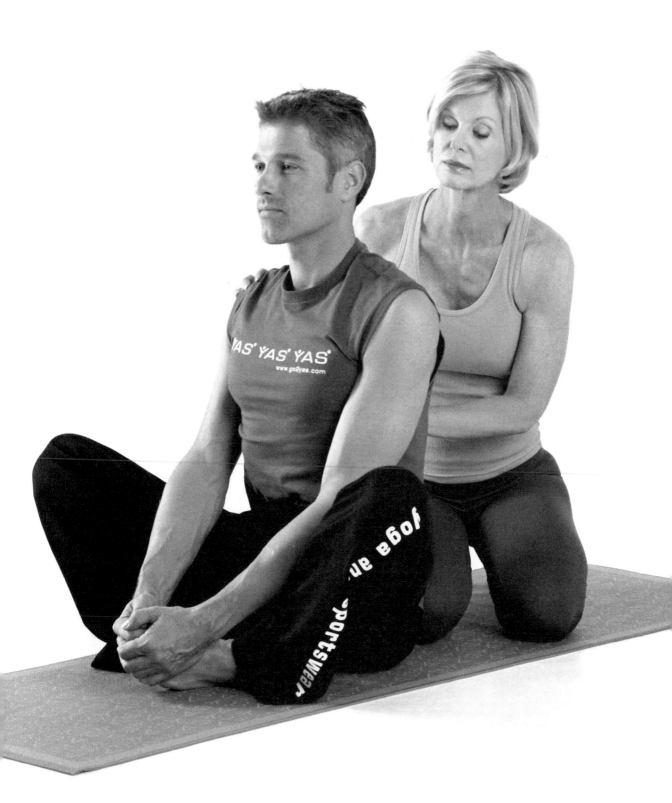

chapter 14

Conclusion

Get off the Couch and on the Mat

If you are inspired to take your first yoga class, which I hope you are, here are some things to know.

QUICK-FIX TIPS

■ It is always good to have a workout buddy. If you have a friend who does yoga, ask him or her to bring you to a class. Make sure you tell your friend it's your first class. You should attend a level 1 or 2 class or a beginner class. "Intro to Yoga" classes can also be a good place to start.

■ Yoga is a barefoot practice, so before you step into the room make sure you take off your shoes and socks.

■ You will need a mat. Call ahead and ask if the studio or gym has mats for you to borrow or rent for a small fee. Make sure you ask how much the rental fee is. You might also have to give them your driver's license if you are borrowing the mat, so make sure you have some ID with you.

- When you get to class, try to be toward the back of the room if possible. I know this seems counterintuitive—most new students want to be in the front row because they think that they will be able to see the teacher better. However, the instructor usually walks around the room, and most don't demonstrate all the poses. In the back you will be able to see and follow the people in front of you.

- You will also need a towel and water. Most studios sell both, but it's always good to be prepared.

- Tell the instructor that it's your first time doing yoga. Don't worry—most studios love to have new students and will make sure they give you extra attention.

- If you have any injuries, tell the yoga instructor before class starts.

- Take a break any time you need to. Just drop down to your mat and come to Child's pose. If you happen to go to a class where the instructor is talking in Sanskrit and chanting, playing a gong, etc., and this makes you feel uncomfortable, get up and leave. This is another good reason to be in the back of the room by the door. Don't feel bad about leaving, and don't give up on doing yoga. There are a ton of yoga studios—you need to find the one you like. If the teacher or the front desk asks why you are leaving, just tell them, "It's not my style of yoga."

What Do I Wear to a Yoga Class?

I constantly get e-mails from people asking me, "Kimberly, what do I wear to a yoga class?" Practically speaking, it will depend on what type of class you are going to. If you are going to a Power Yoga class or a Bikram (Hot) Yoga class, you are going to sweat, so you would want to wear clothes that wick away sweat (similar to what you would wear to go running). Baggy T-shirts are fine for guys, but women should wear a tight-fitting top so that when you are in an inversion (like Shoulder Stand), your top doesn't come down over your head. I often see women trying to pull their tops up in Shoulder Stand because they don't want their stomachs showing—this can be dangerous. Wear quick-dry capri or full-length fitted pants; this will help your instructor check your alignment. Companies such as Lululemon specialize in yoga clothes, but just about every sportswear company has a yoga line at this point. Honestly, you can wear almost anything you would wear to the gym.

There isn't that much "gear" when it comes to yoga; it's basically your mat, strap, and sometimes a block, which most studios provide for you. You also want to bring some water and a towel. As I mentioned earlier, if you are new to yoga and haven't bought a mat yet, call ahead and ask if the yoga studio or gym has mats for you to borrow or rent for the day. I suggest buying your own mat after you have tried a few yoga classes. I find it a little gross to borrow someone else's mat (germs!). Yoga mats come in all kinds of colors and materials, from natural rubber to synthetic, as well as different levels of thickness. I know a lot of books suggest that beginners buy a ¼-inch-thick yoga mat, but that is not such a good idea. It will pad your knees in the floor poses, but when it comes to balancing poses, forget about it! It's really hard to balance on a thick mat. I suggest buying a thinner mat—for one thing, it's cheaper; for another, it will help with your balance. You can always double up your mat for poses, such as Camel, for which you will be on your knees. Use a sponge to wash your mat with soap and water, and let it air-dry.

Most studios provide basic props, such as blocks, which are used to help with alignment, and straps, which can help if you are new to yoga. You can buy your mat at your local sporting goods store or just about any yoga studio. If you want to practice at home, you can purchase mats, straps, and blocks at Web sites such as www.barefootyoga.com and www.yogadirect.com.

Yoga Etiquette

Get there early: Arrive at least 10 minutes before class to get a spot where you feel most comfortable. If you are going to a class that is popular (because of the teacher or the time of day), try to get there 15 to 20 minutes ahead of time. I have students who come to my weekend class a half-hour early to get their spot; they bring the newspaper and read it before class starts.

After you arrive: Take off your shoes and socks before you walk into the room; sometimes studios have cubbies for your shoes, right inside the yoga room. If you are not sure, ask the front desk or just watch what everyone else is doing. As I mentioned earlier, I suggest finding a place in the back by the door. Whether you borrow a mat from the studio or bring your own, make sure you unroll it facing the instructor. I had a student once who came in, placed her mat next to mine, and faced the other students in the class. If you notice that everyone is facing you, you might want to turn around!

Communicate: Before class starts, introduce yourself to the instructor. Tell the instructor whether you have any injury, especially a recent one, so he or she can give you modifications.

Breathe: It's common for new students to hold their breath during yoga poses they find challenging. Breathing deeply can help you relax. In the beginning, don't worry about matching the instructor's breathing instructions exactly; just don't hold your breath.

Practice your basic poses at home: Students at my studios always practice at home. I have a lot of type A personalities, and they want to really "nail the pose." If you practice some of the basic poses at home, such as Downward-Facing Dog, Upward-Facing Dog, Warrior 1, and Warrior 2, which are part of any beginner yoga class, you will feel more comfortable when you do come to class.

Don't leave in the middle of Corpse pose: Most yoga classes end as we do in each chapter of this book, with Corpse pose, also called Savasana (pronounced *sha-vass-ahnah*). With this pose, you lie flat on your back, close your eyes, and relax. You never want to walk out of a class when they are in Corpse pose. If you have to leave, do it before.

Namaste: Don't be scared off when your instructor bows her head as if in prayer, clasps her hands together in front of her heart, and says, "Namaste" (pronounced *nah-mas-tay*). You'll notice the class says it back as well. This Sanskrit word means "I honor you" and is normally said at the end of class.

Types of Yoga Classes

Hatha: This generic term is used to describe any form of yoga that includes physical Asanas (poses). Hatha classes often combine elements from a variety of styles of yoga.

Ashtanga: This form is based on Vinyasa-style yoga, a "flow class" that combines movements with breathing. Ashtanga classes move through six series of poses that increase in difficulty. These fast-paced classes get your heart rate up and build strength.

Power: Power yoga provides a vigorous workout and moves quickly through a series of poses that challenge the core and the upper and lower body.

Iyengar: Poses are held longer than usual in this class; they focus on form and body alignment. Props, from blocks to blankets to chairs, are used. I find this style of yoga great for teachers, but it can be a little tedious for new students. In my first Iyengar class, we spent a full hour on "how to fold your blanket"—oh, man, I could not wait to get out of there! If you have injuries, or if you really want to learn poses, this is a good type of yoga class to look for.

Bikram: Expect to sweat in this class, which is held in 100 degree or hotter temperatures. Bikram is composed of a series of 26 set poses. If you ever get a chance to take one of Bikram Choudhury's classes, you'll find he is quite a character.

acknowledgments

Thank you to Rodale Books for believing in me and helping me get the message out that yoga is for everyone, and not just the few . . . the select . . . the pretzel people.

Thanks, also, to all the students at YAS® Fitness Centers for your continued support, for sharing your stories and allowing me to help you get fit, and for making YAS® the *Cheers* of workout studios and such a rewarding business to own.

I must also thank the thousands of people who have bought my *Yoga for Athletes*® DVD over the years and have used it as part of their training. You, as much as anyone, convinced me that a book like *The No OM Zone* would find an eager audience.

And, of course, my deepest gratitude to my life partner, Sherri Rosen, for her steady support throughout the entire wild ride that has been the bringing of this book to print.

Boldface page references indicate photographs. <u>Underscored</u> references indicate boxed text.